MARKETING

FOR PHARMACISTS

Providing and Promoting
Pharmacy Services
3rd Edition

Notice

The author has made every effort to ensure the accuracy and completeness of the information presented in this book. However, the author and the publisher cannot be held responsible for the continued currency of the information, any inadvertent errors or omissions, or the application of this information. Therefore, the author shall have no liability to any person or entity with regard to claims, loss, or damage caused or alleged to be caused, directly or indirectly, by the use of information contained herein.

MARKETING
FOR PHARMACISTS

Providing and Promoting
Pharmacy Services

3rd Edition

DAVID A. HOLDFORD, RPH, MS, PHD

Professor

Virginia Commonwealth University School of Pharmacy

Medical College of Virginia Campus

Richmond, Virginia

This book is dedicated with love to my parents,
Arthur and Dorothy.

Contents

Acknowledgement: Norman V. Carroll and I have been teaching marketing to pharmacy students for almost 20 years at Virginia Commonwealth University. In addition to his co-authorship of Chapters 3, 4, and 13 of this text, Norm has contributed with feedback and advice throughout the 20 years of teaching this course.

Preface

Marketing for Pharmacists was written for pharmacy students, practicing pharmacists, and pharmacy managers who want a basic introduction to the concepts of marketing pharmacy products and pharmacists' services. This book emphasizes the marketing of pharmacists' services, although it does include some discussion of the marketing of drugs and pharmacy merchandise. The primary purpose of the book is to expose students, pharmacists, and pharmacy managers to techniques and ideas that can make them more effective in meeting the needs and wants of their patients.

Marketing for Pharmacists consists of 15 chapters divided into five sections: Foundations of Marketing, Marketing Strategy, Marketing Pharmacist Services, Consumer Behavior, and Pricing and Marketing Communication. The book is designed to be easily accessible to people without a business background. Nevertheless, it can also benefit those who have substantial experience and training in business.

WHY A MARKETING BOOK FOR PHARMACISTS?

Pharmacy leaders and educators have been telling pharmacists and students for years to challenge the status quo and help forge new professional models within an uncertain, dynamic health care environment. However, pharmacists and students rarely have the experience or training to do so. Their training in basic and clinical sciences does little to prepare them to confront barriers to change. They may be enthusiastic to change pharmacy practice at first, but often their enthusiasm collides with inertia, complacency, and the realities of existing practice. Over time, that eagerness can turn into frustration and helplessness.

Marketing offers a solution for pharmacists. The practice of marketing is a time tested method for bringing about change. It's lessons can be applied to almost any practice related problem faced by pharmacists.

Marketing for Pharmacists was written by a pharmacist as a guide to help pharmacists serve their patients better. It presents the concept of marketing at the level of the individual employee in a hospital or community setting. In contrast, most marketing texts address the topic at the corporate level. The premise of this book is that marketing should be performed by every individual in a business or organization, not just by a corporate department. Pharmacists can use marketing to build their practices, develop and provide innovative services, and generate business for their employers or organizations.

WHO CAN USE THIS BOOK AND HOW?

The book is designed to be used by practicing pharmacists, pharmacy managers, educators, and pharmacy students. Pharmacists and managers can read the book from beginning to end, or they can jump to topics of interest. It is recommended that pharmacists who are not familiar with marketing concepts read the first two chapters, on basic marketing terms and concepts.

Pharmacy educators can use the book, in required or elective courses, to teach students the basics of marketing. *Marketing for Pharmacists* can be used as a text for a broad range of required courses, such as introduction to community pharmacy practice, implementing medication therapy management services, and managing pharmacist services. Alternatively, the book can be used for elective or graduate courses in pharmaceutical marketing.

The chapters cite many references to articles that illustrate the concepts discussed, and readers are encouraged to look for some of those articles. Educators, in particular, can use the referenced articles to supplement information in the chapters and to promote class discussion.

OBJECTIVES

Pharmacists, students, and managers who read this book should gain an appreciation for the need to market pharmacist services and a basic understanding of the principles and terminology of marketing. They should be able to list and discuss important elements of excellent pharmacist services, suggest different methods for designing and providing pharmacist services, delineate processes through which consumers choose and evaluate pharmacy products and pharmacist services, develop a business model or plan, recognize different marketing strategies and understand their advantages and disadvantages, suggest ways to segment markets for pharmacist services, develop a promotional plan, propose innovative pricing tactics not commonly seen in pharmacy practice, and understand marketing channels.

PART I

Foundations
of Marketing

CHAPTER 1

INTRODUCTION TO MARKETING

Objectives

After studying this chapter, the reader should be able to

- Define the term "marketing"
- Explain what it means to have a marketing mindset
- Contrast transactional marketing with relationship marketing
- Discuss some misconceptions surrounding the concept of marketing
- Suggest reasons why pharmacists need to market themselves and their services

A patient tells the pharmacist at a community pharmacy that he would like to quit smoking but does not think he has the willpower to do so. The pharmacist asks several questions to assess the patient's readiness to quit smoking and believes he may be able to quit successfully. The pharmacist encourages the patient to enroll in the pharmacy's smoking cessation program.

A second-year pharmacy student has decided to pursue a residency specializing in community pharmacy. The student knows that community residency positions can be very competitive and wants to maximize her chance of success. She reviews her resume and wonders what she needs to do to gain the right set of skills and experiences to make herself competitive for a residency position.

A hospital wants to open an outpatient satellite pharmacy to serve patients in another part of the metropolitan area. The assistant pharmacy director is asked what services the satellite pharmacy might successfully provide. The assistant director's first step is to identify physicians who practice near the proposed satellite and pay them a visit.

A pharmacist believes her patients would benefit if the pharmacy offered women's health services. However, her immediate supervisor is resistant to change and unlikely to support anything that will make his life more complicated. The pharmacist begins to investigate what resources would be necessary to start a women's health clinic and what strategies might be used to reduce her manager's objections.

The problems faced by pharmacists or future pharmacists in these four scenarios are marketing problems. Pharmacists may label them something else like "career planning" or "clinical practice", but each can be characterized as marketing problems because they involve people trying to satisfy needs and wants. This is the essence of marketing.

This chapter will define marketing and explain its importance to pharmacists and pharmacy students. It will clarify misconceptions about marketing and illustrate different marketing approaches. Finally, it will identify and discuss key problems that pharmacists face in marketing their services.

WHAT IS MARKETING?

Marketing is a process of problem solving, in which marketers attempt to identify and meet the needs of customers. It can be defined as *exchanges between people in which something of value is traded for the purpose of satisfying needs and wants* (Figure 1.1). The key elements of this definition are *people, value, needs and wants,* and *exchange.*

Figure 1.1: The Basic Elements of Marketing

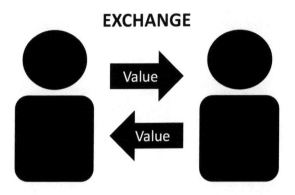

People. Marketing is an act between people. It is a discipline that is interested in human behavior and draws upon the behavioral sciences (e.g., psychology, sociology, and anthropology). Marketers want to know why people act the way they do and how they can be influenced. Some might question the labels given to individuals in transactions like "marketer" and "customer" or "consumer". The term marketer implies that marketing is something inflicted on customers, when it is really just a process of serving the other party in a transaction. The terms customer and consumer suggest someone who passively consumes what is produced by the marketer, but today, they are actively engaged in communicating their needs, helping co-produce value, and sharing their experiences with others.

Value. Marketing deals with transactions of value. The items of value do not necessarily have to be money or tangible products. Indeed, marketing increasingly consists of exchanges of intangible information, ideas, and wealth. Google and Facebook are some of the largest companies in the world, but they offer intangible products in exchange for information about you and your networks. Items of value in transactions can be anything that might meet a need or want, including money, material, labor, information, and ideas.

Needs and wants. Marketing is concerned with satisfying the needs and wants of individuals. Needs are things that people must have to survive, such as food, water, clothing, transportation, and shelter. Wants are things that are desired but not absolutely essential for survival. People often confuse needs and wants. A person may say that he "needs" a Mercedes-Benz automobile, but he is really saying that he wants one, since the need for transportation can be met in many other ways. The person who says he needs a Mercedes-Benz is really expressing a preference or want for one specific mode of transportation over another.

Exchange. For the process of marketing to occur, there must be an exchange or the potential for an exchange between two of more individuals. Without an exchange of something of value, needs or wants cannot be satisfied. Ideally, this exchange should benefit everyone involved. In an exchange in a pharmacy, the pharmacist and patient both give something and get something. If both sides are satisfied afterwards, the exchange is a success.

> *It's all marketing.*
>
> *—Anonymous*

MARKETING EXCHANGES

There are two ways of looking at marketing exchanges. The first is to look at exchanges as isolated, individual transactions that involve people who never expect to do business again. The second is to see exchanges as a series of transactions over time. How a marketer looks at exchanges helps determine how he or she practices marketing.

Marketers who view exchanges as isolated and unrelated events are practicing *transactional marketing*. In transactional marketing, the goal of each party is to maximize the benefit received from each transaction. In every exchange, it is important to drive a hard bargain, because there is one opportunity to maximize the value received. Since the parties do not expect to ever do business again, there is no concern about future exchanges, partner customer satisfaction, or customer loyalty to the business.

An alternative approach is to see exchanges as a series of transactions over time. Parties using this approach, called *relationship marketing,* see each transaction as an opportunity to develop and strengthen a long term relationship with the customer. Relationship marketing focuses less on bargaining hard for deals and more on meeting the needs of the other party. The goal is to have transactions in which both parties are satisfied, because satisfaction can lead to future business. Relationship marketers attempt to cultivate relationships over time, because they believe the long term benefits will be greater than the benefits of transactional marketing.

Pharmacists have been moving from a transactional to a relationship marketing approach to serving patients and customers. It is no longer possible to succeed in business by completing the sale and getting the patient out the door of the pharmacy. Now, pharmacists need to view each customer interaction as one step in the process of building a long-term relationship with that customer. Each occasion to speak with a patient, physician, nurse, or other person is an opportunity to establish or strengthen a relationship.

For example, a pharmacist can view the act of telephoning physicians to make therapeutic recommendations as a single event or a series of events over time. A pharmacist with a transactional viewpoint is only concerned with completing the call and getting on with other work. The outcome of the call is less important than the desire to conclude it as quickly as possible.

With a relationship viewpoint, the objectives for the telephone call change. The first and most obvious objective is to get the physician to accept the recommendation. A second, less obvious objective is to establish or maintain the pharmacist's credibility as a source of future therapy recommendations. Even if the physician does not accept the pharmacist's immediate recommendation, the pharmacist has laid the groundwork for acceptance of future recommendations. Pharmacists who practice relationship marketing take each exchange seriously, realizing that one bad interaction with a patient or health care professional can hurt future ones.

EVERY PHARMACIST IS A MARKETER

When we take the broad view that marketing consists of exchanges of things of value between people, it becomes clear that any activity directed toward meeting people's needs and wants is a marketing activity. Accordingly, pharmacists who engage in any of the following actions are involved in marketing:

- o Dispensing a prescription drug,
- o Assisting patients in the selection of nonprescription medications,
- o Providing drug information to patients or health care professionals,
- o Taking a patient's blood pressure,

- Counseling patients about drug regimens,
- Convincing key decision makers of the benefits of pharmaceutical care,
- Recruiting pharmacists for a new job, and
- Educating pharmacy students.

With this broad definition of marketing, nearly everything pharmacists do in their jobs is a marketing activity. Therefore, to be successful in pharmacy, pharmacists need to be good marketers.

Marketing is about influencing others. It is finding out what people need and want and getting them to take actions to meet those needs and wants (e.g., make a purchase, take their medicine as directed). Marketing pharmacy services is about influencing the following people:

Patients. Pharmacists persuade patients to take their medicines as directed, use nonprescription medicines appropriately, follow instructions, monitor their therapy, and pay for a higher level of services.

Physicians. Pharmacists influence physician behavior through persuasive conversations and written communications.

Third-party insurance companies. Pharmacists try to persuade third party insurance companies to pay higher dispensing fees and reimburse pharmacists for professional services.

The pharmacist's employer. Pharmacists induce employers to hire them over the many other pharmacists competing for a job. Once in a position, pharmacists continually try to demonstrate their value to their employer.

The pharmacist's boss. Pharmacists encourage their bosses to manage differently, try new ways of meeting the needs of patients, and maximize rewards for good work.

The pharmacist's co-workers. Pharmacists influence co-workers when they sell them on new ideas, get them to participate in group projects, and motivate them to handle a fair share of the workload.

MARKETING IN ACTION

Branding Yourself

Every year, students graduate from pharmacy school with enthusiasm and relief. Most find high-paying jobs that meet all of their physical needs. However, many find that their chosen career paths do not meet their emotional and/or intellectual needs. Why?

In most cases, it is simply because they have been passive in developing and managing their careers. Rather than systematically looking for and crafting an engaging career and life, they choose to let random events and others control their life.

Indeed, successful careers are built on a lot of luck. But successful pharmacists enhance their career chances by marketing themselves and their personal brand.

A Pharmacist's Personal Brand

Branding is the process of developing strong, positive, and consistent images of your brand in the minds of people who interact with the brand. Your name is your own personal brand. Your name will conjure up an image in the minds of people with whom you interact (e.g., professionalism, competence, responsiveness). The stronger and more positive those images, the better your relationships will be with people.

The strength of your personal brand is determined by the extent that people (1) recognize your name when they see it and (2) recall it when making a choice. The more familiar and memorable your name, the more likely people will think of you. And the more positive and consistent the image associated with your name, the more credibility you will have in the minds of people.

Some people are lucky in their personal brands by having unique and memorable names. In high school, my art teacher was named Mrs. Artsner. After students verified that her name really was Mrs. Artsner, they remembered it. Few people had to be told her name twice.

People with common names, like David, have more difficulty getting people to recall their brands. They have to work harder to establish and maintain clear, positive associations with their personal brand in the minds of colleagues and others.

Developing the Right Mindset

The key to marketing yourself is to have a positive and healthy attitude toward promoting yourself and your career. Marketing yourself is not about bragging or making yourself out to be something you are not. Rather, marketing is about trying to find the right opportunities for you. This process includes:

- *Understanding yourself* – What do you want? What is important to you?
- *Knowing your target customers* – With whom do you want to work? What do they need and value in coworkers? What problems do your customers need solved?
- *Developing a clear value proposition* – What unique value do you provide to your work and career relationships? What solution do you provide for your customers?
- *Identifying and sizing up your competition* – Who are you competing

with for career opportunities and professional relationships? How do you match up to what they have to offer?

- ○ *Building a network of partners* – Who supports your career? Who are your mentors, collaborators, and letter of recommenders? What are you doing to make it easier to support you?
- ○ *Researching the market* – What kinds of careers are available for you? What is the daily work like? How do different careers meet your personal and professional needs?
- ○ *Communicating your message* – What do you want others to know about you? How can you promote your ability to help them and provide value to their work?

Packaging Your Brand

Everything you do or say reflects on your personal brand, so it is important to pay attention to how you present yourself to others. Understand the image you project in how you behave with classmates, coworkers, professors, friends, and family. Your actions, words, and body language will communicate some message. Ask yourself if that is the message you want to send.

Both your personal life and professional life can affect your brand. Be consistent in both arenas. A misstep in one can hurt your image in another. A bad personal reputation can easily impact your professional image. Some recommendations:

- ○ Dress professionally. If you are in doubt about what to wear, overdress. You can always take a suit jacket off or remove your tie if you are too formally dressed for the occasion.
- ○ Learn to use a strong handshake. A limp handshake sends a message of weakness and insecurity.
- ○ Make eye contact when you talk to people.
- ○ Have an up-to-date resume or CV readily available.
- ○ Have business cards made up and keep them in your wallet or purse.
- ○ Have a positive social media presence. When people conduct an internet search of your name, make certain that something comes up that is consistent with your brand.
- ○ Remember people's names. If you learn their names, they will be more likely to remember yours.
- ○ Take care in how you write to others in e-mails and letters. A poorly worded phrase or sentence can come back to bite you.
- ○ Be nice to everyone even if they can do nothing to promote your career. How you treat individuals who can do nothing for you sends a strong message.

WHY MARKETING IS IMPORTANT TO PHARMACISTS

Marketing is too important to be left to the marketing department.
David Packard, Co-Founder of Hewlett-Packard

Given the changing demand for pharmacists and the increasing prescription workload, the prospects for pharmacists are not completely clear. The U.S. health care system has limited resources to manage the nation's health. Health care providers (e.g., physicians, nurses, hospitals, managed care organizations) are all competing for a portion of those resources. Providers who demonstrate and promote their value are more likely to thrive in the future health care environment.

No one knows what the future will bring to the pharmacy profession. All we know is that things are going to change. The ability to market oneself and one's practice is a way for pharmacists to adapt to changes in health care. There are tremendous opportunities for pharmacists who are willing to market themselves and their professional practices.

PHARMACIST SKEPTICISM ABOUT MARKETING

Some pharmacists and pharmacy students are skeptical about the relevance of marketing for pharmacists. Often, this skepticism results from misconceptions about marketing. Many people think of marketers as unethical people who intrude into your life, clutter the landscape with advertising, and interrupt your favorite television and radio shows to try to get you to buy things that you really don't want. In truth, marketing is often practiced that way. However, not all marketing is like that. For example, marketing is used to:

- o Increase vaccinations for deadly diseases
- o Promote medication therapy management to skeptical patients
- o improve the image of pharmacists and pharmacist services
- o Reduce demand for antibiotic use for treating colds and viral infections
- o Influence compliance with prescribing guidelines
- o Help patients adhere and persist with their medications
- o Aid new graduates in finding their ideal job

Many tasks in health care are the same as tasks in marketing - they just have different names (Table 1.1). "Health care" is called "serving customers" in marketing; "managing a professional image" is called "branding"; "motivational interviewing" is very similar to what marketers call "personal selling", and so on. In fact, there are few terms in health care that do not have matching marketing labels.

Table 1.1. Matching Marketing and Health Care Terms

Health Care Term	Marketing Term
Patient	Customer or Consumer
Health Care Provider	Producer, Marketer
Health Care	Serving Customers
Health Care Environment	Market
Epidemiology	Market Research
Patient Needs Assessment	Marketing Research
Health Communications	Promotional Communications
Health Care System	Marketing Channels
Professional Image	Brand
Patient Centered Care	Personalized Service
Motivational Interviewing	Personal Selling
Medication Therapy Management	Relationship Marketing

MISCONCEPTIONS ABOUT MARKETING

A person may ask, "Why do I need marketing? I am a pharmacist (or will be one soon). I don't want to be some fast-talking used-car salesman. I want to save lives and improve patients' quality of life, not peddle my services to customers. Besides, pharmacy is a health care profession. It has a higher purpose and is above the need for (ugh!) marketing. Besides, I plan to work in clinical pharmacy, where marketing is not important. If not, I'll work for an employer who will handle all that marketing stuff for me. Marketing has very little applicability to my current or future practice."

The following misconceptions about marketing are common among pharmacists and pharmacy students:

1. *Marketing is selling.* Selling is just one function associated with marketing. Other marketing functions include researching customer needs and wants, developing strategies, maintaining customer records, delivering products and services, financing, promotion, pricing, and monitoring customer satisfaction. Selling is completing a sale. Marketing covers the sale and all of the activities before and after the sale.

2. *Marketing is bad.* Some critics charge that marketing is inherently bad because it results in socially undesirable actions such as overconsumption, waste, and the purchase of products that people would do better without (e.g., cigarettes). Although it is accurate to say that marketing can promote socially negative acts, it is also true that marketing can be used to promote positive behaviors. Marketing has been used to promote AIDS prevention, smoking cessation, birth control, and other preventive health behaviors. Although we may dislike the marketing of some products (e.g., liquor and cigarettes), marketing can benefit society.

3. *Health care professionals do not need to market.* If you look at successful health care professionals, be they physicians, nurse practitioners, optometrists, dentists, or pharmacists in any setting, you will see that they excel at marketing. They may just call it something else.

4. *Employee pharmacists in community pharmacies do not need to market.* Most employee pharmacists have a great deal of autonomy in how they practice, with relatively little oversight from their bosses. In many cases, these pharmacists are responsible and held accountable for the success of their practice sites. Upper management may provide support services such as TV or newspaper advertising or research about the local market, but in the end, most marketing in pharmacy is conducted by individual pharmacists through the services they provide and the personal relationships they develop with their patients.

A basic premise of this book is that all pharmacists can use marketing as a tool to help others. Like any tool, marketing can help when used appropriately and hurt when misused.

DEVELOPING A MARKETING MINDSET

Pharmacists need to develop a new mindset to thrive in the changing health care environment. The old mindset will not need to necessary changes in practice. A pharmacist's mindset determines how problems in practice are approached and determine how patients benefit. The old mindset for pharmacy practice is illustrated by approaches like the production, product, and expert approaches (Table 1-2).

Table 1-2 Approaches to Marketing

Approach	Driving Force	Philosophy
Production	Efficiency and Speed	Be fast and cheap
Product	The product idea	If we build it, they will come.
"I'm the expert"	Expert opinion	I know what is best for you.
Modern marketing	Needs and wants of customers and society	How can I help you? How can we make the world a better place to live?

Production Approach. The production approach to marketing holds that the major task of any pharmacy or pharmacist is to pursue efficiency in production and distribution of medications and services. Success occurs when the pharmacy runs smoothly. The assumption is that cheap and efficient provision of goods and services is sufficient for success in business. With this approach, there is little explicit consideration of the needs and wants of patients and society. The assumption is that if products and services are cheap enough, customers and society will demand them.

A pharmacy that takes a production approach to the provision of services may attempt to fill as many prescriptions as possible, without consideration of whether consumers benefit from the prescriptions. Such a pharmacy treats patients not as individuals but as units of production; the more units that travel through the process, the better. With this approach, pharmacies compete almost entirely on the basis of price and availability. But the fact that something is produced and available does not mean that it will be wanted and purchased.

Price and availability may not be a sustainable strategy if there is someone cheaper and more accessible. Decades ago, independent pharmacists who competed solely on price were underpriced by chain pharmacies that were able to take advantage of economies of scale. The pharmacies that have survived learned to compete by offering something more than low price and convenience. The lesson to be learned is that low price and availability are often not sufficient for survival in the market.

Product Approach. With the product approach, pharmacists become so passionate about a product or service that they are blind to its need and market viability. The problem is that high quality products may be more than what is needed or wanted. The philosophy of the product approach is, "If you build it, they will come." This can cause a narrow-mindedness that leads pharmacists to place the needs of the product over the realities of the market.

Not to be confused with the production approach, the product approach assumes that a business that develops a better product will automatically find consumers who will buy it. But even the best products on the market can fail. They can be too expensive, poorly promoted, difficult to find and purchase, or of higher quality than customers need or want.

Some pharmacists have taken a product approach to marketing medication therapy management (MTM). As originally designed, MTM consists of five core elements: medication therapy review, a personal medication record, a medication-related action plan, intervention and referral, and documentation and follow-up.[1] Although anyone who uses medications can benefit from MTM, many enthusiastic pharmacists have been dismayed about weak demand for it. To benefit and thrive, MTM may need to evolve to better meet the realities of the health care market.

"I'm the Expert" Approach. This approach occurs when pharmacists believe that they know better than patients what is best for them. It expects customers to comply with the directions and guidance of pharmacists. It contrasts with patient-centric care where the patient is more involved in deciding what is best. The "I'm the expert" approach often overlaps with the product approach to marketing. Both are paternalistic; they do not include the patient in decision-making. Health care professionals often take this approach because they think their many years of education make them more qualified to decide a patient's treatment. Modern health care is moving away from this approach but it is still common.

Modern Marketing Approach. The modern marketing approach asserts that the main task of an organization is to determine the needs and wants of targeted customers and satisfy them through the design, communication, pricing, and delivery of appropriate and competitive products and services.

This approach has several distinguishing features. First, in designing, promoting, and delivering products and services, it explicitly considers the viewpoints of customers. This means that the customer drives decisions about marketing strategy—not the product, provider, or production. Second, modern marketing focuses on targeted customers; marketers match their products and services to those customers whom marketers can serve better than their competitors can. Targeting recognizes that circumstances do not necessarily support every idea and venture, so marketers need to focus on meeting the needs of select customers. Finally, the modern marketing approach seeks to satisfy customers and relevant stakeholders.

Still, this approach does not blindly pursue satisfaction of the primary customer, because other Individuals and institutions may have a stake in the outcome. The modern marketing approach takes responsibility for the consequences of marketing practices on society - recognizing that satisfying some people can hurt others. An extreme example is trying to satisfy a drug addict which may mean giving the addict drugs on demand. Although it satisfies the addict in the short term, it may not be in the best interest of either society or the drug addict over time. Similarly, patients may be satisfied with fast, cheap, and friendly service from a pharmacist, but if that service does not help them adhere to their medicine or avoid negative health events, it would be hard to conclude that a pharmacist's service is providing real value to the patient or society.

From this point onward, this book uses and advocates for the modern marketing approach in pharmacy practice. When pharmacists adopt this approach in serving patients, payers, and other stakeholders, they can satisfy the needs and wants of their immediate patients, profession, and society.

PROBLEMS ASSOCIATED WITH MARKETING PHARMACIST SERVICES

It would be wonderful if the public recognized and fully appreciated the contributions of pharmacists - and equally wonderful if pharmacists could practice in the manner promoted by the profession. However, pharmacists function in the real world, where the practice of pharmacy is constrained by a number of realities. Some of the realities that must be overcome before pharmacists can reach their full professional potential are described in the following sections.

Control of Practice by Nonpharmacists

Unlike many other professionals in the United States, pharmacists have limited control of how their profession is practiced. Pharmacist control over the profession has gradually decreased as corporate ownership of pharmacies has increased. In the past, pharmacy ownership was limited to licensed pharmacists; today, most pharmacies are controlled by corporate entities. These corporations are answerable to shareholders and often are run by nonpharmacists.

With corporate ownership, the primary job of pharmacy managers is to enhance shareholder value. Therefore, corporate managers make decisions based on profit, a framework that is not always consistent with the goal of enhancing patients' health and well-being. When a pharmacist must choose between filling prescriptions (which generates revenue) and counseling or therapeutic problem solving (neither of which generates revenue), it is easy to see the conflict.

Nonpharmacist owners are also less likely to fully appreciate the problems associated with inappropriate drug use. They lack the training, experience, and professional socialization required to fully grasp many of the issues facing practitioners of pharmacy. Nonpharmacist owners are likely to be distracted by nonpharmacy concerns within the business. Prescription drugs are only a small portion of the overall business in many large corporations, especially mass merchandisers and grocery stores. Corporate owners may consider the practice-related concerns of pharmacists to be of minor consequence.

Product Orientation

Most pharmacists in the United States work in community pharmacies that use a retail business model. The retail business model revolves around selling merchandise. Service is a major component of retailing, but the success or failure of retail businesses ultimately depends on the sale of tangible goods.

The product focus of the community pharmacy model contrasts with the professional service model found in medicine, law, and other professions. The professional service model is typically oriented toward information and counseling. Revenue is generated from these activities. This contrasts with the retail business model, in which revenue comes from providing a broad range of merchandise for customers in a convenient manner.

In recent years, changes have been seen in many community pharmacy settings to emphasize the professional nature of pharmacists and the value they provide. Pharmacist employers recognize a need to increase revenue streams in areas like increasing medication adherence, reducing drug related problems, offering vaccinations, and providing clinical services. Outcomes research and published report cards on the quality of pharmacist services may speed up the move from an orientation that focuses on drugs to one that emphasizes the outcomes associated with those drugs.

Conflicting Professional and Merchant Roles

The pharmacy profession and pharmacists must often struggle to balance their professional and merchant roles. Pharmacists are responsible for making a profit as well as for helping patients with their health-related needs. This balancing act can cause conflict.

Pharmacists must generate revenue by filling more prescriptions. Time that is not spent filling prescriptions (e.g., time spent on patient counseling and disease management activities) does not usually generate revenue. However, pharmacists have a professional responsibility to monitor patient therapy, educate and counsel patients, and solve therapeutic problems even if no revenue is generated. These are the professional activities that can truly improve patient health and quality of life. Most pharmacists continue to face this struggle daily.

Poorly Defined Public Image of Pharmacists

Although the public's image of pharmacists is generally favorable, most consumers do not have a clearly defined image of what a pharmacist does. Ask a person on the street what a pharmacist does, and the person is likely to say something vague about dispensing medicines. It is unlikely that the person will know anything about the details of the tasks involved in dispensing or the pharmacist's role in medication therapy management. This lack of awareness can lead to low expectations of pharmacists and little recognition of the value they provide.

A Potential Oversupply Supply of Pharmacists

In the second edition of this book, there was a concern about pharmacist shortages. That problem has been resolved and then some. Since 2000, the number of pharmacy schools in the US have increased 60% and expanded student enrollments in older schools have lead to a 70% increase in the annual number of new graduates.[2] Concerns have arisen that an oversupply of pharmacists may lead to joblessness and underemployment.

The looming oversupply of pharmacists can impact the marketing of pharmacist services in unpredictable ways. It may lead to a shakeout where only the best pharmacists survive in the job market - weeding out pharmacists who are unwilling or unable to provide exceptional MTM and other clinical services. It may also have a positive impact by reducing complacency and entitlement of some pharmacists and increasing their willingness go the extra mile for their patients and employers. Downward pressures on salaries may make pharmacists more affordable alternatives to physicians and nurse practitioners in primary care settings. On the other hand, it may make pharmacists so fearful about losing their jobs that they place employer concerns before those of patients, even if doing so is unethical or unprofessional. Only time will tell.

MARKETING IN ACTION

CVS Bans One-Stop Shopping for Prescriptions and Cigarettes

CVS took a big step recently toward becoming a health care company by removing tobacco products from its shelves in late 2014. Its decision to ban sales of tobacco products coincided with a company rebranding of its corporate name to CVS Health (CVS), from CVS/Caremark Corp. This step was taken to reflect the company's broader health care commitment and desire to change the future health of Americans.

This decision was not made without consequences to the retail business. It was estimated that CVS Health would lose $2 billion in annual sales of tobacco products.

Nevertheless, the move was hailed by public health leaders, providers, insurers, and payers. The public relations benefit of the decision has been viewed as a boon to the CVS brand. It has also clearly differentiated itself from competing retailers who still sell tobacco such as Walgreens and Wal-Mart.

Source: Reference[3]

SUMMARY

Pharmacy marketing is not just about selling drugs. It is also about promoting new ideas. Marketing can further the idea that pharmacists provide value and should receive compensation for professional services. It can help pharmacists exert influence over the way pharmacy is practiced.

Marketing can be used to solve almost any problem in pharmacy. It can be used in personal career management, in influencing change in practice settings, and in enhancing job effectiveness. Marketing can help persuade patients to adhere to medication plans, physicians to prescribe medicines appropriately, and management to support pharmacy practice initiatives. It can be used to recruit good employees, attract and keep patients, provide innovative services, and compete with other professions for a portion of the health care pie.

This book focuses on marketing ideas and methods that can be used by pharmacists. It is based on the premise that marketing is not just a corporate activity but an activity that needs to be practiced by every pharmacist.

Reference List

(1) Medication therapy management in pharmacy practice: core elements of an MTM service model (version 2.0). J Am Pharm Assoc (2003) 2008;48(3):341-353.
(2) Brown DL. A looming joblessness crisis for new pharmacy graduates and the implications it holds for the academy. Am J Pharm Educ 2013;77(5):90.
(3) Japsen B. CVS Stops Tobacco Sales Today, Changes Name To Reflect New Era. Forbes [September]. 9-3-2014.

Exercises

1. List specific examples of how marketers have intruded into your life, irritated you, or deceived you. Compare those with examples of how marketers have made your life better. What differentiates the "bad" marketers from the "good" ones?

2. Think about a pharmacist or fellow student who you believe has an excellent reputation. What behaviors does this person engage in to develop such a positive image? Would you consider this person to be a good marketer? Why or why not?

3. Will Rogers, famous cowboy philosopher, has been quoted as saying, "Let advertisers spend the same amount of money improving their product that they do on advertising, and they wouldn't have to advertise it." Do you agree or disagree with this? Why?

4. How might pharmacists use marketing to
   a. Enhance their personal career opportunities?
   b. Provide better care for patients?
   c. Promote a positive image of pharmacists among the public?

5. What major barriers do pharmacists face in providing clinical services such as diabetes management in your practice setting?

6. List things of value that are exchanged between pharmacists and patients, physicians, and nurses.

7. Describe what you think are the greatest barriers to the progress of the profession. Discuss how these barriers can be overcome.

Activity

Identify an issue in the professional pharmacy literature or on a professional association Web site that might be marketing related. Describe the issue and why you think it relates to marketing.

CHAPTER 2

IMPORTANT MARKETING CONCEPTS

Objectives

After studying this chapter, the reader should be able to

o   Define key marketing terms: product; core, expected, and augmented product; marketing myopia; potential, target, and actual markets; the marketing mix; the four P's; positioning; value proposition; service-dominant logic
o   Explain the difference between customers, partners, and competitors
o   Describe two major categories of competitors
o   Differentiate internal from external customers
o   Describe the "products" offered by pharmacists
o   Identify and differentiate the various marketing tasks, the type of demand they regulate, and suggested strategies

This chapter discusses some basic marketing concepts—product, customers, competitors, and market—that pharmacists need to understand to market their services.

MARKETING IN ACTION

Lina's Dilemma

Alfreds is a discount department store chain that recently entered the market in the Mid-Atlantic States. This regional chain has 125 stores in 12 states. Forty of the stores have pharmacies, and more pharmacies are planned for the next 2 years.

Alfreds advertising literature describes a customer-friendly attitude: "We consider our customers to be our guests." Alfreds tries to provide high quality products at low prices. The stores offer a wide range of merchandise, including snack bar items; school and office supplies; stationery and party favors; hardware; apparel for men, women, and children; small appliances; jewelry and accessories; home decorating supplies; housewares and commodities; health and beauty aids; candy and snack foods; cameras and electronics; pet supplies; prescription and nonprescription drugs; bathroom accessories, bedding, window treatments, and rugs; and furniture and lighting. The stores are well-lighted and convenient, and service is fast and friendly.

One metropolitan area has five Alfreds stores, the first of which opened in April 2000. Each of these stores has a pharmacy that provides basic dispensing services and vaccinations on-demand. Alfreds' management wants these five stores to start providing medication therapy management (MTM) services to provide new revenue to supplement declining dispensing profits. Alfreds and a local school of pharmacy have reached a collaborative agreement to promote the practice of MTM in the area. Alfreds will fund a full-time clinical faculty member from the school to oversee the implementation of MTM in each individual store and to create quality advanced practice experience rotation sites for PharmD students.

The faculty member, Dr. Lina Kennedy, wants the Alfreds initiative to have a major impact on patient care. Her success in the effort hinges on effectively marketing the MTM program to Alfreds customers, employees, supervisors, and other interested parties.

Dr. Kennedy was asked to develop a business plan for her initiative that answers a variety of questions including:

1. What product will the program be offering? What value proposition will she be making to her customers?

2. Who are Lina's potential customers, partners, and competitors?

3. What is the market for MTM in the geographic area served by Alfreds? How can she expand the product over time?

DEFINING THE PRODUCT

In the factory we make cosmetics; in the drugstore we sell hope.
—Charles Revson, founder of Revlon Cosmetics

The average person thinks of products as tangible objects that are sold for and bought with money. Examples include automobiles, computers, furniture, clothing, and drugs.

Marketers define the term more broadly. A concise and widely recognized definition of a *product* is "anything of value that can be exchanged to satisfy a need or want."[1] According to this definition, a product can be an object (e.g., a syringe of antibiotic), a service (e.g., cholesterol screening), an activity (e.g., a poison prevention campaign), a person (e.g., Bob, the clinical pharmacist), a place (e.g., a Medicine Shoppe pharmacy), an organization (e.g., the American Pharmacists Association), or a concept (e.g., medication therapy management). Each is valued and satisfies needs or wants. For example, Bob, the clinical pharmacist, offers solutions to the needs of his employer and the patients he serves. The American Pharmacists Association offers benefits to its members and the profession as a whole.

How pharmacists define their product is critically important, because it specifies the ultimate purpose of pharmacists and frames the way in which they approach pharmacy problems. The defined product shapes pharmacist priorities and actions. If pharmacists define their product as the provision of a drug, they fit the "count and pour, lick and stick" and "pill pusher" labels that some people associate with pharmacists. These pharmacists practice a production approach (see Chapter One) to marketing, in which they focus on the provision of a tangible product (i.e., a physical object).

However, people pay for the benefits of drugs, not the tangible drug product. Patients, insurers, and other purchasers pay for the positive health outcomes that drugs can bring, such as pain relief, quick recuperation from illness, reduced risk of death, and improved quality of life. The tangible drug is just a vehicle for delivering health benefits associated with the drug.

Drugs by themselves rarely bring about health benefits. Indeed, a patient can be harmed if she does not know how to take the drug appropriately. Pharmacists who fixate on the provision of a tangible drug suffer from what marketers call marketing myopia. *Marketing myopia* is shortsightedness on the part of marketers who become preoccupied with selling the tangible product while failing to consider the needs of the consumer.[1] Marketing myopia exists when pharmacists see themselves as providers of drugs rather than managers of drug-related health outcomes.

To prevent marketing myopia, the *total product concept* was introduced.[1] This concept (Figure 2-1) looks at a product in terms of three primary components: (1) the core product, (2) the expected product, and (3) the augmented product.

Core Product

The *core product* (center circle in Figure 2-1) is the benefit resulting from the bundle of tangible goods, information, and services offered to the customer. It meets the underlying need that the overall product package satisfies. It is what the customer is really buying. The woman who purchases a camera is not buying a mechanical box; she is buying pleasure, nostalgia, and a form of immortality.[2] The middle-aged man who buys a sports car is not buying a means of transportation; he is buying memories of youth and the hope to relive them. For customers of pharmaceutical services, the core product may be health related (e.g., improved quality of life) or not (e.g., greater peace of mind, a feeling of control over one's illness).

Figure 2-1 Total Product Concept

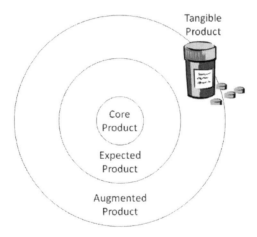

It must be emphasized that the core product is defined by the consumer—not the marketer—because the consumer is the only one who can assess whether an underlying need has been satisfied. For example, the benefit of a health care intervention program may be better health, peace of mind, control over a health condition, or any other number of benefits. The marketer can only identify the core product when the consumer reveals it, typically through marketing research surveys, focus groups, in-depth interviews, and observation.

Pharmacists often mistakenly assume that the core product patients seek is health; this is not always the case. A man undertaking a prostate screening may not be seeking avoidance of disease but peace of mind. A woman may not really have realistic expectations that she will be able to achieve long-lasting weight loss; she may just be in search of hope that it might happen. Understanding the core benefit sought is critical for every element of a marketing mix. Therefore, assumptions about the benefits sought in engaging in healthy behavior should be questioned and verified.

Some marketers have re-framed the idea of core products into the concept of *jobs-to-be-done*.[3] They argue that success in business comes from a deep understanding of the job the customer is trying to accomplish. Patients who buy a drug or visit a pharmacist are hiring a solution to a problem. The key to innovating in pharmacy is to identify jobs the customer needs to get done and develop solutions for them.

The best known example of jobs-to-be-done was described by Clayton Christenson in an anecdote labeled "milkshake marketing." In this example, Christenson observed that people who visit fast food chains in the morning often purchase milkshakes to be consumed during their morning commute.[4] Puzzled because milkshakes are not considered breakfast food by most people, he interviewed purchasers about why they bought milkshakes. His conclusion was that milkshakes were being hired to give commuters something to do on their drive and to hold off hunger until lunchtime. That insight was used to increase morning milkshake sales among commuters.

The jobs-to-be-done framework encourages pharmacists to think about the job from the customer's perspective by asking "What job is the patient trying to get done?" For patients, the job of purchasing a prescription medication may consist of several jobs like acquiring the medication, fitting the medication into one's daily routine, and self-monitoring. Each job can be an opportunity for the pharmacist.

Expected and Augmented Products

The next circle in the total product concept is the *expected product*. The expected product is what the customer expects to receive from a marketer. The expected product is situation specific; it varies according to the circumstances and the people involved. When dispensing drugs in a pharmacy, the patient may expect only to receive the correct drug in an accurately labeled container within a reasonable time period. In other circumstances, the expectation may be higher or lower.

Anything provided that is beyond what the customer expects is called the *augmented product*. The augmented product is the bundle of tangible product(s), information, and services that exceeds the customer's minimal expectations. The augmented product is also called the differentiated product because it differentiates one business from the next. Things that might augment community pharmacy services include counseling, therapeutic monitoring, insurance assistance, free home delivery, blood pressure monitoring, refill reminders, telephone and Internet refills, selection of nonprescription medications, patient package inserts, compliance programs, drive-through services, and disease management services.

The expected product and augmented product provide a bundle of benefits that result in the core product. A pharmacy's bundle of services and merchandise is meant to fulfill patients' health care and non-health care needs. The more a patient perceives the benefit bundle as unique and valuable, the more likely it is that the patient will patronize the pharmacy.

In reality, no bundle of services and merchandise offered by any pharmacy is exactly like any other (e.g., no two pharmacies are likely to be equally convenient), although the patient may perceive pharmacies as interchangeable. How a pharmacy differentiates its product from those of competitors determines the relative value to the patient. If a pharmacy wants to attract and keep patients, its differentiated product should offer greater value in their eyes.

MEASURING THE MARKET

To the average person, market refers to a physical place where buyers and sellers gather to exchange goods and services. To a marketer, the term *market* means the set of all individuals and organizations who are actual and potential buyers of a product or service. A market consists of anyone who might conceivably buy a given product.[1,5]

A market includes actual and potential buyers. Actual buyers are current customers. Potential buyers are people or groups who might have (1) a real or unrealized interest in products or services and (2) the means to acquire them. By this definition, wherever there is potential for trade, there is a market.

For many products, the potential market is only a fraction of the overall population within a given area. This is not the case in pharmacy, because the majority of people in the US consume medications. Since anyone who consumes pharmaceuticals may also benefit from monitoring, counseling, and drug information, the potential market for MTM care is quite large.

Within the potential market are the target market and the actual market. The target market consists of those people in the potential market who are deemed most attractive to the marketers. These people might be targeted because they are most profitable or best suited to the capabilities of the marketer. The target market is the focus of marketing efforts.

The actual market is those people who actually consume products or services. It is typically much smaller than the target market and may even include individuals outside the target market. Its size depends on how successful a marketer is in attracting and keeping customers within a market. The actual market for products depends on the customer's:

1. Level of interest. Customers must be aware of a product and recognize a need for it.

2. Necessary resources. Customers must be able to pay for the product.

3. Willingness to pay. Customers must be willing to pay for the product.

For higher levels of pharmacist services such as MTM, the target and actual markets are likely to be smaller than the potential market. The target market is smaller because some patients may not currently need intensive pharmacist services and because providing such services may not be profitable, given the lack of compensation by prescription drug insurers. The actual market for these services may be further limited if people are (1) unfamiliar with the availability and features of MTM, (2) unaware of their need for it and how they might benefit, (3) unwilling to pay for it, or (4) unable to pay for it.

Therefore, for MTM to achieve its market potential, pharmacists must Identify people in the population who might benefit from MTM (i.e., the potential market), Identify and attract people in the potential market who best match the services that pharmacists can provide (i.e., the target market), and serve those customers who have sufficient interest and resources to pay for it (i.e., the actual market).

THE MARKETING MIX

The term *marketing mix* describes the actions that can be taken by marketers to attract and keep customers. The marketing mix is popularly known as the four P's of product, price, promotion, and place. Businesses compete with each other by offering some combination of product, price, promotion, and place designed to cause customers to choose their product over a competitor's.

The product is the array of tangible goods, services, and information offered, as described earlier in this chapter. The price is what is asked of customers in exchange for the product. Promotion refers to communications designed to inform, persuade, and remind customers about the product. Place is the manner, location, and ease of access to the product.

The marketing mix for a prescription drug consists of elements of the four P's that differentiate one pharmacy from another. Table 2-1 lists elements of the marketing mix associated with the dispensing of a prescription drug. To address unique elements of the marketing mix associated with services, some service marketers have expanded the four P's to seven P's.

The three extra P's associated with services are physical evidence, participants, and process. Physical evidence refers to the physical environment in which services are provided and all tangible cues (e.g., employee dress, documentation, and signage). Physical evidence is related to place; it includes elements associated with the location of the service, such as the parking lot and physical building. Participants are all personnel associated with the provision of services, including both providers and customers. Participants are related to product and promotion. Process includes all policies, procedures, rules, guidelines, and workflow design associated with the provision of services. Process is most closely related to product.

An additional P, positioning, is mentioned by some marketers. *Positioning* refers to the development of a favorable image in the minds of customers. The position of a product in the mind of the customer is determined by virtually anything the customer sees, hears, smells, tastes, and touches relating to that product. The product itself and how it is priced, promoted, and delivered determine its image in the mind of a customer.

Although the extra P's of physical evidence, participants, process, and positioning may help draw attention to factors of importance to marketers, all of them can be viewed as falling within the traditional four elements of the marketing mix. Therefore, for the sake of simplicity, this book describes the marketing mix in terms of the original four P's: product, price, promotion, and place.

VALUE PROPOSITION

The marketing mix summarizes the total value being offered by a pharmacy. When making a decision to purchase or act on the offering, customers weigh what they have to give with what they receive. The price to the patient in terms of money, time, effort, and other costs is compared with impressions about the quality, benefits, convenience, expertise, and support being offered by the pharmacist. In essence, the pharmacy or pharmacist is making a persuasive argument to customers. Marketers call this the *value proposition*.

A value proposition is a promise to customers of the value to be delivered in exchange for some price. It explains in a compelling and clear manner why a product or service solves a problem or makes things better for customers than competing options. Good value propositions convince customers that what is being offered is worth every penny and ounce of effort being asked.

To create a value proposition, pharmacists need to know several things. One is the specific audience which often varies depending on the target audience. For instance, a value proposition for a diabetes management clinic might differ for diabetics, the physicians treating those diabetics, an employer who is insuring diabetics, and a PBM who wants to control diabetic drug costs. Another thing that must be known is the problem(s) faced by customers for which a solution is offered (e.g., non-adherence with medications, uncontrolled warfarin levels, lost productivity of employees due to health related problems).

Based upon that information, the value proposition presents the main features of the value package to be provided (e.g., The medication adherence program consists of a five step process that...) and how it compares with other options in the marketplace (e.g., There are few programs designed for improving medication adherence in area and ones which are available do not..."). Finally, the value proposition can be supported by evidence or logic-- called *proof points*. An example of a proof point is, "A study in the New England Journal of Medicine found that similar program was 20% more effective than the standard of care."

A good value proposition clearly, concisely, and powerfully articulates the unique value of a service or product to targeted customers. They often evolve over time. As more is learned about the customer, the proposition can be fine tuned to more effectively appeal to targeted audiences.

IDENTIFYING COMPETITORS AND PARTNERS

Competitors

In most circumstances, pharmacists compete with others to serve customers. It is rare for a pharmacist or pharmacy to have a monopoly on the market, so it is important to identify competitors. Once identified, these competitors need to be challenged in the market. Awareness and understanding of competitors is crucial, because all elements of the marketing mix are assembled with an eye toward these competitors.

Identification of competitors requires a clear definition of one's market or markets. Pharmacists and pharmacies often serve multiple markets. Community pharmacies might serve the prescription drug, cosmetics, photographic, and convenience food markets, as well as many others. A pharmacy's competitors for the prescription drug market may be different from its competitors for the other markets.

Competitors can be divided into two categories.[1] Those in the first category, *intratype competitors*, compete by providing the same or similar products. Examples of intratype competitors in the automobile market are General Motors and Ford. Examples in fast food include McDonalds and Burger King. In community pharmacy, Walgreens, Rite Aid, and CVS are intratype competitors.

Those in the second category, *intertype competitors*, compete by providing distinctly different products that nevertheless meet similar customer needs and wants. Examples of intertype competitors in the evening entertainment market include cinemas, television, restaurants, and local sporting events. Each offers a completely unique product to meet the entertainment needs of consumers. Examples of intertype competitors in other markets include airline and railroad travel, mail and Internet communication, and pharmaceuticals and complementary medicine.

Intratype competitors compete by offering similar tangible and augmented products. They are more immediate threats than intertype competitors, because they compete openly and directly for customers. Intratype competitors are likely to be perceived as substitutes by customers, which makes competition for customers more acute.

Intertype competitors compete in terms of the benefits provided (i.e., the core product). Although they are less likely to be perceived as substitutes, they are still competing. In fact, intertype competitors can be more dangerous, because it is easier to overlook them. IBM failed to see the competitive threat personal computers (PCs) posed to its mainframe business because it did not see PCs as direct competition.

An often overlooked competitor for pharmacist services is the status quo or inertia (i.e., resistance to change). When pharmacists offer a clinical service designed to help patients, they must realize that patients can always decide to do nothing or continue doing what they have always done. Doing nothing is typically easier and free.

Not changing (i.e., not using the clinical service) requires no additional effort or expenditure of money. Even pharmacist services that are fully covered by a patient's health insurance still require time and effort by the patient. To compete with the status quo, the pharmacist must convince patients that participating will be worth it.

MARKETING IN ACTION

Social Marketing

Social marketers view competitors differently from commercial marketers.[6] Commercial marketers see competitors as anyone who might contend for customers' dollars. *Social marketers* seek to improve the social welfare of individuals and populations, so they view competitors as anything that gets in the way of socially desirable behaviors.

Social marketers in health care consider their primary goal to be health, not profits. They see their stiffest competition as unhealthy alternatives to healthful behaviors - not other health care professionals or businesses. For this reason, pharmacists who adopt a social marketing approach to health promotion might view other pharmacists employed by business competitors as social marketing allies.

The primary competitor of social marketers is existing unhealthy behavior. Existing unhealthy behavior is a tough adversary because it is often habitual, maybe even enjoyable. Little effort is needed to continue with unhealthy, pleasurable habits - unlike healthy behaviors which may require effort and expenditures of money. Consequently, to persuade people to change, social marketers must lay out a clear value proposition that offers convincing reasons to change.

Other important competitors to behavioral change are the various opponents of healthy behavior whose self-interest conflicts with healthy behaviors. For instance, tobacco companies compete with smoking cessation programs for the hearts and minds of cigarette smokers. These companies engage in massive advertising and public relations campaigns to counter the messages offered by opponents of smoking. Any marketing program for influencing healthy behavior must develop counterstrategies to opponents of change.

Source: Reference [6]

To understand their competition, pharmacists need to know how their product is perceived by customers. As shown in Table 2-1, the way the product is defined determines who the competitors are. Pharmacies whose product is perceived as "filling a prescription" have different competitors from those whose product is defined as "part of a lifelong process of managing patients' health."

Table 2-1 Relationship of Competitors to Product Definition

Product Definition	Competitors
Filling a prescription	CVS, Walgreens, Rite Aid, Kroger, Wal-Mart, independents Dispensing physicians Robotic dispensing machines Mail order and Internet pharmacies
One step in a process of purchasing household products, groceries, and prescription drugs	CVS, Walgreens, Rite Aid, Kroger, Wal-Mart, independents 7-Eleven, Quickie Mart Any other general merchandise store without a pharmacy Mail order and Internet pharmacies
Part of a lifelong process of managing patients' health	CVS, Walgreens, Rite Aid, Kroger, Wal-Mart, independents Physicians, nurses, and other health care professionals Health food stores and providers of complementary medicine Mail order and Internet pharmacies

Partners

In health care, potential competitors can become partners through strategic alliances or other forms of partnerships. Strategic alliances occur when two or more parties agree to pursue together mutually beneficial objectives while remaining independent of each other. A collaborative practice agreement is a form of strategic alliance.

Pharmacists can partner with other pharmacists, physicians, nurses, local businesses, employers, health systems, PBMs, insurers, professional associations, wholesalers, local pharmacy schools, governmental entities, and pharmaceutical companies to serve patients. If partners are able develop arrangements to work together, they and the patient can benefit.

Partners need to be cultivated inside and outside of the organization. Outside partners can offer resources, information, access to patients, or other help. But an often overlooked category of partners are individuals within the pharmacy organization. Key internal partners include management, technicians, clerks, store manager, other pharmacists within the organization, and support staff like those in information technology and billing. Engaging internal partners is often critical to the success of pharmacy initiatives.

MARKETING IN ACTION

Who is the Customer?

Defining the primary customer of pharmacists services is often difficult because health care has so many people involved in the decision making process, and their roles vary depending on the circumstances. Typical roles in health care are:

- Influencer - An individual whose advice can change some element of the buying decision
- Decider - The person with the authority to make the ultimate decision regarding purchase
- Patient - The person who actually consumes the product or service
- Provider - The individual or organization who provides a particular product or service
- Producer - The individual or organization who produces a particular product or service
- Payer - The one who pays for all or part of the health care product or service
- Care Provider - A friend or family member who provides care to a patient

In some situations, these roles are filled by a single individual - cash purchase of a nonprescription medicine for personal use. In other cases, the roles overlap like when a provider of MTM services also acts as a producer and influencer. The following example illustrates the various roles in a single health care visit.

A child's mother (influencer) notices that the child appears ill and tells her husband to take the child to the doctor. The husband (decider) chooses to take the child to their pediatrician for care. The child (patient) is prescribed an antibiotic by the pediatrician (provider). The prescription is taken to the pharmacist (provider) which is filled with a medication that came from a pharmaceutical company (producer). The patient is covered by a health insurer (payer) who pays the pharmacy for the drug and the dispensing fee. Each day, the mother (care provider) administers the antibiotic to the child as prescribed.

The challenge for marketers is to understand all of the participants in a health care decision and the roles they play. This will be necessary to effectively serve the ultimate consumer.

CUSTOMERS OF PHARMACIST SERVICES

Who are the customers of pharmacists? They include not just those who come into the pharmacy, but anyone with whom pharmacists must deal. By this definition, everyone who interacts with pharmacists can be considered a customer.

The External Customer. External customers are the people outside your organization with whom you deal, either face-to-face or over the telephone. They include customers in the traditional sense of the word: the people who purchase your products and services. External customers also include your suppliers, the general public, and anyone else you might interact with outside the organization. Interactions with external customers determine the image of your organization. They can also influence the quality of your product, because external customers are often participants in the provision of services. Imagine trying to encourage patient adherence to medication regimens without patient participation.

The Internal Customer. Your other customers are the people who work inside your company and rely on you for the services and information they need to do their jobs. They are not traditional customers, yet they need the same levels of service that you give your external customers.

This point was brought home to me when I was a pharmacist at a hospital that was attempting to improve the quality of services we provided. We were asked to identify the customers of our pharmacy department. Customers were defined as anyone with whom we had dealings either inside or outside the hospital. One of the things we found is that we did not treat some of our internal customers (e.g., housekeeping and engineering personnel) with the respect that should be accorded a customer. We did not greet them when they came into the pharmacy and often treated them as if they were not even there. When pharmacy personnel started to acknowledge their presence with a "Hi" or "Is there anything we can do to help?" the pharmacy employees found that these simple acts led to better communication with those departments and resulted in much better service for the pharmacy and its external customers.

MARKETING TASKS

Although the process of marketing consists of many activities, the ultimate task of marketing is to influence demand. Marketers influence demand for their products and services through their use of marketing tools such as promotional communications, price, and service. Marketers influence demand in a way that helps achieve specific marketing objectives.

This does not always mean increasing demand.[5] Many times marketers want to decrease demand or keep it steady. Different situations in which pharmacists or other health care marketers can influence demand are described in Table 2-2.

TABLE 2.2 Marketing Tasks

Market Demand	Description	Health Care Examples	Recommended Marketing Strategy
Negative Demand	When potential customers dislike a product and may even go to great lengths to avoid it.	Screening for colon cancer even when at high risk. Men's aversion to vasectomies, concern about vaccinations, and fear of needles and dental work.	Understand the dislike in order to overcome it. Negative demand might come from misconceptions that may be overcome by education or peer-to-peer counseling. In other cases, interventions might need to address complex social or psychological beliefs.
No Demand	When customers are indifferent or uninterested in a product.	Preventive health care services and MTM services.	Stimulate interest in the product; possibly by connecting the benefits of the product with a person's needs and interests.
Latent Demand	When there is a strong need but no product available to satisfy it.	There are unmet needs for cures for cancer, effective and easy-to-take weight loss pills, affordable health care insurance for everyone, and drugs without adverse effects.	Fill latent demand by (1) identifying unmet demand, (2) assessing its extent in the marketplace, and (3) developing innovations to fulfill those unmet needs.
Declining Demand	When demand is falling and likely to continue falling. Most products eventually reach this phase where they eventually decline and die.	The old time pharmacy - a meeting place where people could get their prescriptions filled, have a drink at the soda fountain, and chat with friends.	Rejuvenate demand by improving the product itself, repackaging it in a new and appealing manner, or promoting it to untapped market segments. Some pharmacists have successfully revitalized their pharmacies by tapping into people's nostalgia for the old time pharmacies of their childhood.
Irregular Demand	This describes a market with undesirable fluctuations in demand.	Retail pharmacy practice where customers decide the time and place to visit their pharmacists.	Use a variety of strategies to even out demand over time. These include the use of technology, redesign of pharmacies, promotion of special senior citizen discount days, and scheduling of appointments.
Full Demand	A highly desirable situation in which supply is perfectly balanced with demand.	Good examples are uncommon because it is rare to successfully balance supply and demand over time.	Balance supply and demand by working hard to maintain high quality, keeping current with the changing desires of customers, and defending markets against competition.

| Overfull Demand | When demand exceeds supply. | Drug shortages due to unexpected demand situations or shortages in supply. | Either increase supply or reduce demand in an acceptable manner. Common strategies include increasing production, raising prices, lowering quality, or reducing convenience. |
| Unwhole-some Demand | Demand that is not in the best interests of the consumer or society. | Cigarette, illicit drug, and underage alcohol use | Paint the product as something undesirable. For example, the messages "Smoking kills" and "Smoking is not cool" may be used to discourage adolescents from smoking. |

SUMMARY

Knowing marketing terminology helps pharmacists learn marketing concepts. There are important lessons in the use of specific terms. For example, a discussion of intratype and intertype competitors teaches that competition originates not just within one business category or profession; rather, it can arise from any business that seeks to fill the same core needs as your business. Knowing marketing terminology can help pharmacists in speaking with business managers. Most people with a rudimentary business background know and use these terms. An understanding of these terms is necessary background for the later chapters in this book, which explain more complex marketing concepts.

Reference List

(1) Levitt T. What business are you in? Classic advice from Theodore Levitt. Harv Bus Rev 2006;84(10):126-37, 150.

(2) Hibbard JH, Greene J. What The Evidence Shows About Patient Activation: Better Health Outcomes And Care Experiences; Fewer Data On Costs. Health Affairs 2013;32(2):207-214.

(3) Christensen CM, Baumann H, Ruggles R, Sadtler TM. Disruptive innovation for social change. Harv Bus Rev 2006;84(12):94-101, 163.

(4) Christensen CM, Cook S, Hall T. Marketing malpractice: the cause and the cure. Harvard Business Review 2005;83(12):74.

(5) Kotler P. Marketing Management: Analysis, Planning, and Control. 4th ed. Engelwood Cliffs, NJ: Prentice Hall; 1980.

(6) Holdford DA. Marketing of Pharmacy Health Promotion Programs/Activities. Health Promotion and Maintenance. Pharmacotherapy Self-Assessment Program (PSAP). Sixth ed. Lenexa, KS: American College of Clinical Pharmacy; 2008. 118-132.

Exercises

1. Define the core, expected, and augmented product marketed by
   a. Your pharmacy to patients.
   b. A pharmacy professional association of your choice to potential members.
   c. You to potential employers.
   d. A pharmacy school to students

2. Describe the difference of medication therapy management and basic dispensing services to a friend of family member. Share the problems you faced in doing so.

3. List the internal and external customers of your pharmacy.

4. List the intratype and intertype competitors of your pharmacy.

5. Give one example of a product or service for which you personally have each of the following:
   a. Negative demand
   b. No demand
   c. Latent demand
   d. Declining demand
   e. Irregular demand
   f. Full demand
   g. Overfull demand
   h. Unwholesome demand

CHAPTER 3

MARKETING CHANNELS
Co-authored by Norman Carroll

Objectives

After studying this chapter, the reader should be able to

- Describe what are marketing channels and their functions in pharmacy practice
- Summarize the arguments for and against using intermediaries in channels
- Map out general pharmacy channel structures
- Identify the sources of channel conflict
- Suggest strategies for managing conflict in marketing channels
- Define key terms: channels, intermediaries, just-in-time, outsourcing

This chapter discusses marketing channels and their value in pharmacy practice. Channels within the health care value chain are covered. This chapter explores more than channels of distribution which stress a product-centered approach to marketing channels. Rather, it discusses a broad range of channels and their functions in pharmacy with the goal of broadening the understanding of what pharmacists must do to serve their customers.

MARKETING IN ACTION

Next Day Delivery? Try Next Hour!
Next-day delivery may soon be too slow for pharmacists and pharmacies. Next-hour shopping is rapidly approaching as a standard option for receiving medications and other health care products. Retailers like Walmart and Amazon are testing same-day delivery services for all types of merchandise; from ice cream to flat screen televisions. They are doing this by revamping their marketing channels with software that rely on complex computational algorithms, human and robot workers who man enormous distribution centers 24/7, and even door-to-door delivery drones.

Walmart used to rely on *just-in-time delivery*— the science of making merchandise available on shelves right before it is needed by a customer. Using a vast hub-and-spoke system, their 158 distribution centers could serve its 4,000 some stores, quickly and efficiently. However, to compete with online retailers like Amazon, they have started using some stores as forward-deployed inventory centers that act as mini-warehouses for local delivery. Employing algorithms to track 1.2 million transactions per hour, Walmart is able to track the movement of goods and anticipate what stores will need to serve the demands of home-delivery shoppers. This is how a delivery from WalMart works.

1. Noon: Shop at Walmart.com/togo for a product that is locally stocked.

2. 1 PM: The order is filled at one of the stores/mini-warehouses. A picker, robot or human, pushes a wheeled rack down the aisles, placing items in blue bins.

3. 2PM to 4PM: Walmart trucks are loaded with items to be delivered.

4. 4PM to 8PM: Walmart delivers to your door.

One can easily see delivery drones replacing Walmart trucks for prescription orders. Drones give the ability to fill and deliver orders within an hour. One small company in the San Francisco area, quiqui (Pronounced Kwi-Key) is reported to already be offering drone delivery of prescriptions to your door.

This means that pharmacies will face increasing pressures to speed deliveries to customers. Same-day, even same-hour delivery, might be needed. Brick-and-mortar pharmacies are going to have to offer something that online retailers cannot. Pharmacists will need to step up their service to give customers a reason for coming inside a physical store.

Sources: References[1, 2]

Pharmacists are important to effective medication use, however, they just one of many links in a chain of channel providers serving individuals' medication related needs. Wholesalers, manufacturers, pharmacies, health insurers, regulatory agencies, financing organizations, and other channel members are links in the value chain for pharmaceuticals. Each creates additional value by providing essential functions to receive the benefits of drugs. The more value each channel member contributes, the more profitable and successful it is likely to be in health care.

MARKETING CHANNELS

Marketing channels are the paths through which goods, information, and payment travel on their way from the producer (e.g., manufacturer) to ultimate consumer (e.g., patient). In pharmacy, there are channels for distributing medications, financing and paying for those medications, insuring risk associated with medications, and facilitating their appropriate use. Channels of distribution are a prominent concern for pharmacists.

A *channel of distribution* consists of the producer of a good (e.g., drug), the ultimate user, and any intermediaries (i.e., middlemen) through which the goods pass. A typical channel of distribution for a medication consists of the manufacturer (e.g., Merck or Pfizer), a pharmaceutical wholesaler (e.g., McKesson or Cardinal), a community pharmacy, and the patient who ultimately receives the medication (Figure 3.1). Other channels of distribution may have fewer or more intermediaries.

Channels are made up of interdependent entities that work to serve customers. Channels exist whenever an intermediary exists between a producer and buyer. The basic structures of marketing channels are shown in Figure 3.2. They can consist of one seller and many buyers, one buyer and many sellers, or a combination of sellers and buyers.

Figure 3.1 Example of a Pharmaceutical Product Channel

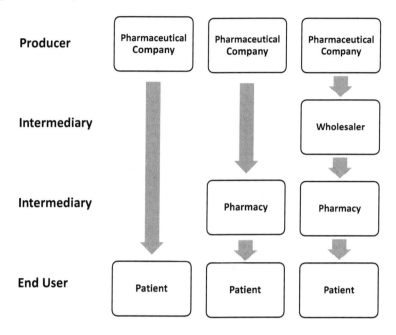

Intermediaries improve the efficiency of distribution channels by decreasing the number of required interactions between members of the channel. A simple example shows how this works. Assume that a distribution channel consists of three buyers and three sellers. If each buyer makes a transaction every day, then 9 interactions (3 times 3) are required per day. Four buyers and sellers require 16 transactions per day, five buyers and sellers require 25, and so on. When multiplied by 365 days per year, the number of transactions can be enormous. However, when one intermediary is introduced into the channel between sellers and buyers, the number of total daily transactions drops from 9 to 6; the number of contacts for each buyer and seller drops to 1.

Figure 3.2 Basic Marketing Channels

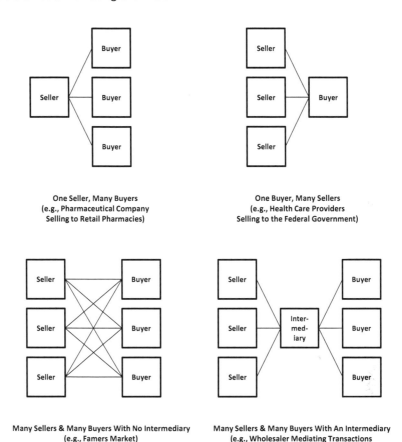

One Seller, Many Buyers
(e.g., Pharmaceutical Company
Selling to Retail Pharmacies)

One Buyer, Many Sellers
(e.g., Health Care Providers
Selling to the Federal Government)

Many Sellers & Many Buyers With No Intermediary
(e.g., Famers Market)

Many Sellers & Many Buyers With An Intermediary
(e.g., Wholesaler Mediating Transactions
Between Pharmaceutical Companies and Retailers)

Producers benefit from working with channel intermediaries in several ways:

1. Intermediaries offer platforms which can be used by large numbers of producers in an economical way. Multiple pharmaceutical companies can use one wholesaler to serve thousands of pharmacies. Instead of dealing with thousands of pharmacies, the pharmaceutical company only needs to deal with one wholesaler. Similarly, a pharmacy only needs to deal with one wholesaler instead of numerous drug companies. This reduces the number of transactions needed and reduces channel costs.

2. Intermediaries reduce the amount of upfront investment required by producers. For example, a new biotech company can more quickly and cheaply

put a drug on the market by hiring marketing firms, sales management companies, wholesalers, and other intermediaries to serve diverse functions instead of doing it on its own. Indeed, some pharmaceutical firms are virtual, consisting solely of a small team of individuals which contract all operational tasks associated with the development of promising drug candidates.[3]

3.   Specialization of intermediaries adds quality and efficiency to the system. Wholesalers, pharmacies, PBMs, and other intermediaries focus on a limited number of tasks which they do better and more cheaply than any other chain members.

4.   Specific skills and capabilities can be efficiently outsourced to channel partners. *Outsourcing* is defined as the contracting of some function associated with a business that would otherwise have been provided by the firm itself.[4] It is based upon the premise that all tasks that can be done cheaper or better elsewhere in a channel should be outsourced. For example, insurance companies employ pharmacy benefit managers (PBMs) to manage the millions of pharmacy transactions that occur in pharmacies. PBM investments in infrastructure and systems allow them to serve this function more efficiently than anyone else in the value chain.

CHANNEL FUNCTIONS AND FLOWS

In addition to channels of distribution, there are many other marketing channels that facilitate the work of moving services and products. They perform some of the following key functions:[5]

- o   Storage of physical goods
- o   Financing the movement of goods and services
- o   Assuming financial risks connected with work in the channel
- o   Developing and providing promotional communications
- o   Collecting and interpreting information collected by channel partners
- o   Managing regulatory affairs and relationships with key parties

Some functions are associated with the flow of physical goods; others with the flow of money, communication, information, and services. Flows can go forward to the end user (e.g., drug) or backward to the producer (e.g., payment). Each intermediary in the channel serves one or more functions (Figure 3.3).

Figure 3.3 Marketing Channel Functions

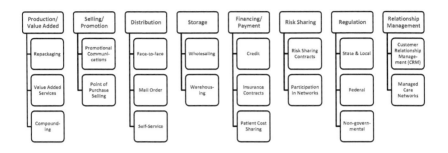

PHARMACEUTICAL CHANNEL MEMBERS

Marketing channels for pharmaceuticals and pharmacist services are much more complex than that seen in other industries. This complexity is due to the fact that the end consumer is not usually the only decision-maker. One of the most important decision makers is the physician who acts as an intermediary by prescribing drugs and having final authority over what gets prescribed. Other important intermediaries in health care include health insurance companies, pharmacy benefits managers, pharmacists, government regulators, and others. A variety of entities are involved in the medication use channel including the ones described below.

Pharmacies

The primary role of pharmacies is medication use control. They are intermediaries between physicians, pharmaceutical manufacturers, third party payers of pharmaceuticals, and insurers of medication use. There are many types of pharmacies including community, hospital, clinic, long term care, specialty, mail order, and internet pharmacies.

The overall value provided pharmacists and pharmacies in marketing channels are often masked by the complexities of the health care system. Pharmacists are typically seen as distributors of drugs when they may also serve other non-distributive functions including advising, selling, promotion, storage, risk sharing, regulation, and relationship management. Examples of the functional roles that pharmacies and pharmacists may serve in channels are illustrated in Table 3.1.

Table 3.1 Marketing Channel Functions and Examples of Pharmacists Roles

Channel Function	Example of pharmacist role
Production & Adding Value	Providing MTM & clinical services
Promotional Communications	Persuading patients to adhere to medications
Distribution	Dispensing medications
Storage	Inventory & formulary management
Financing & Payment	Assisting patients & providers in cost effective therapeutic plans
Risk Sharing	Managing risk of adverse outcomes of medications
Regulation	Ensuring that all other channel members adhere to laws & regulations
Relationship Management	Developing & maintaining therapeutic relationships with patients

Services provided within pharmacy channels can be synchronous or asynchronous. *Synchronous pharmacy services* are defined as those which are produced and received at precisely the same time. Examples of synchronous services are face-to-face interactions between a pharmacist and a patient or a person-to-person phone call.

Asynchronous services are those which can be produced and stored in electronic media like web pages, videos, and other forms, typically mimic the length of channels for physical goods. Asynchronous services are most commonly seen in web-based communications or educational materials. This might include informational webpages, online self assessments, informational webinars and broadcasts, and more.

A typical channel of distribution for an asynchronous pharmacy service consists of the producer (e.g., a pharmacist or pharmacy organization), an electronic media platform (e.g., Youtube or LinkedIn), a media consumption device (e.g., computer or smart phone), and the consumer who ultimately receives the product.

Synchronous services differ from asynchronous services in ways that can affect their delivery and influence how they fit within marketing channels. Since synchronous services are produced and received at precisely the same time, they cannot be stored for later distribution and use. This leads to discrepancies in service supply and demand. A pharmacist in a community pharmacy might have too few customers one moment and too many the next. If some of those services can be offered asynchronously (e.g., interactive video recording), service supply and demand might be evened out. The disadvantage of asynchronous services is that they do not offer the human element of synchronous services. No matter how well designed an asynchronous service, an engaging interaction face-to-face with a well trained pharmacist will offer something that an interactive video or website cannot provide.

Manufacturers

A *manufacturer* is a business that produces a finished product from raw materials. Examples of pharmaceutical manufacturers are Merck, Pfizer, and Barr Laboratories. The pharmaceutical industry has two basic types of manufacturers: research oriented and generic companies.

Research-oriented manufacturers not only manufacture drug products, they also conduct research to discover and develop new drugs. The Pharmaceutical Research and Manufacturers of America (PhRMA) is the trade group representing the research oriented manufacturers. Details about its members can be found at its website www.phrma.org.

A growing sector of the research-oriented pharmaceutical industry is biotechnology. These companies are represented by the Biotechnology Industry Organization (BIO) which lists details about its members at www.bio.org . Some research intensive companies are members of both PhRMA and BIO.

The second type of manufacturer is the generic drug company. *Generic drug companies* manufacture products that are no longer protected by patents. They spend relatively little on research and development. Generic drug companies outnumber research-oriented companies, but they are much smaller organizations. Details about this industry can be found at the Generic Pharmaceutical Association (GPhA) website at www.gphaonline.org.

Wholesalers

A *wholesaler* is a business that purchases finished goods for resale to other businesses. Wholesalers do not sell to ultimate consumers. In the past, pharmaceutical wholesalers limited their function to purchasing prescription and nonprescription products from manufacturers and selling them to pharmacy retailers. Large wholesalers like AmerisourceBergen, Cardinal Health, and McKesson have expanded their businesses to include functions including distribution of medical and surgical products, operating networks of independent pharmacies and radiopharmacies, business consulting, inventory management, business process assistance, various technology services, medication packaging, specialty pharmacy services, group purchasing organization networks, and more. The Healthcare Distribution Management Association (HDMA) is the trade group representing pharmaceutical wholesalers (www.healthcaredistribution.org).

Health Care Insurers

A *health care insurer* is a company that sells health insurance policies to individuals or sponsors (e.g., employers who offer insurance to employees). *Health insurance policies* are contracts in which the insurer accepts the financial risk of negative health consequences to individuals in exchange for the payment of periodic premiums. For example, an individual may wish to insure himself or herself from the risk of large expenses due to unexpected illness or trauma. That individual can purchase an insurance contract from an insurer where the individual agrees to pay monthly premiums in exchange for the insurer paying some or all of the costs of health events like hospitalizations or long term care. Many individuals are covered under group insurance contacts where sponsors (e.g., employers, government) pay premiums.

Examples of insurers include Wellpoint, Kaiser, Aetna, and Humana which act as intermediaries between patients and health care providers. These health care insurers contract with providers (e.g., pharmacies) to serve policy holders' needs. To reduce their risks and potential costs, insurers try to influence the quantity and quality of health care by requiring providers to agree to certain terms in contracts. For instance, pharmacies might sign contracts to substitute generic medications for brand name medications, meet certain patient satisfaction scores, and accept low dispensing fees.

Pharmacy Benefit Managers

Pharmacy benefit managers (PBMs) manage the pharmacy benefit for health care insurers acting as an intermediary with physicians, pharmaceutical manufacturers, and pharmacies. PBMs develop and maintain formularies of drugs that will be covered and under what conditions those medications can be used. PBMs also process and pay prescription drug claims, sign contracts with pharmacies to be in networks to service insured individuals, and negotiate discounts and rebates with pharmaceutical manufacturers. Some PBMs have expanded into the provision of care by offering mail order pharmacy services.

State, Federal, and Local Governments

Government is involved in all functions of marketing channels. The U.S. government is one of the largest purchasers of health care including prescription medications. As major purchasers of medications and services, they establish many rules and regulations which influence all aspects of pharmacy practice. This ranges from research, development, and manufacturing of medications (Food and Drug Administration) to payment and delivery of care (Medicare, Veterans Administration). State and local governments are also heavily involved in marketing channel functions. State Medicaid programs regulate many aspects of delivery of and payment for care. State regulatory bodies also directly influence channels by licensing pharmacies and pharmacists (state boards of pharmacy).

The role of government in pharmacy marketing channels is so extensive that any discussion is beyond the scope of this chapter. There is very little about the practice of pharmacy which is not directly or indirectly influenced by government involvement.

CHANNEL RELATIONSHIPS

Marketing channels consist of different organizations, each with their own goals and objectives. In pursuing their goals, organizations frequently find themselves in conflict with other organizations in the channel. At other times, they may cooperate with the other organizations to reach mutual goals.

Channel Conflict

Figure 3.4 illustrates some of the relationships between pharmaceutical channel members and the primary function each serves within the channel. Conflict is inevitable when members fulfill their basic functions. For example, when the Federal and State governmental agencies perform their regulatory functions, they conflict with members involved in insurance, prescribing, and distribution who will generally resist attempts to constrict their ability to serve their customers.

Conflict can increase when channel members try to take on new roles that compete with other channel members. Some physicians bristle at pharmacists who take on new practice responsibilities like administering vaccinations, providing disease management services, and offering anything related to traditional physician roles. Conflicts between pharmacies and PBMs have increased as PBMs moved beyond benefit management to dispensing of medicines through mail order operations. The potential for conflict will occur when any channel member gets in the way of another member achieving its goals.

Some conflict is good. Conflicts are needed to disrupt the status quo and lead change in health care. They can also help enforce desirable behaviors in channel members who may otherwise act in illegal, unethical, or uncompetitive ways. For instance, government regulation helps protect consumers and the public from physical and financial risks in the marketplace. Competitive conflicts between channel members can improve provided services and help ensure better value for customers. The key to managing channel relationships is to ensure that any conflicts remain productive.

When unproductive conflict between channel members occurs, it impairs the efficiency and effectiveness of the channel. For example, some channel conflicts have solidified the status quo. Conflicts between community pharmacists and opponents have hindered pharmacists' ability to gain provider status (so far). Lack of provider status has hindered pharmacists' ability to engage in medication reconciliation and offer other solutions to inappropriate medication use.[6] Conflicts have occurred with PBMs that develop restricted pharmacy networks which limit access of some pharmacy providers to patients.

Figure 3.4: Primary Pharmaceutical Channel Relationships

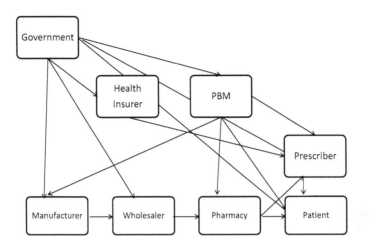

MARKETING IN ACTION

Conflicts in Pharmacy Networks

Conflicts between pharmacy benefits managers (PBMs) and Pharmacies are often in the news. Walgreens has been prominent in many because they have butted heads with the PBMs Express Scripts and CVS' PBM Caremark.

The first conflict occurred when contract-renewal talks between Walgreen Co. and Express Scripts Inc. broke down over reimbursement rates for filling prescriptions. Stated simply, Express Scripts told Walgreens to accept the reimbursement rates offered or lose access to customers whose prescriptions were insured by the PBM. Walgreens thought that Express Scripts would never want to lose access to Walgreens' thousands of pharmacies, so they refused the low rates. The PBMs surprised Walgreens by shutting them out of their pharmacy networks and sending business to Walgreens' competitors.

Over the next year, Walgreens saw significant reductions in prescriptions filled and front-end store sales. Eventually, they had to give in to Express Scripts reimbursement demands after losing millions of dollars in the conflict.

A second conflict was related to CVS Health's move to stop selling tobacco products. The pharmacy chain gave up an estimated $2 billion in annual sales from tobacco products in their retail stores to rebrand themselves as a provider of health care, not a retail business.

To make up some of those lost sales, CVS Health's Caremark PBM announced that they would charge an extra co-payment (up to $15) at any pharmacies selling tobacco products. This move was seen as controversial because it would give CVS retail pharmacies an advantage over competitors who still sell cigarettes, including Walgreens and many independently owned pharmacies. Critics of the plan saw it as a blatant move to inhibit competition for pharmacy customers. Furthermore, it appeared that CVS Health implemented the plan primarily to help its CVS retail business and Caremark PBM and damage competitors.

CVS responded that the decision was a health issue, not an issue of competition. They stated that Caremark clients asked for "tobacco-free" pharmacy networks, and that tobacco use was one of the most common causes for morbidity and mortality in the world. They argued that the move was to save lives.

The conflict over this issue was not yet resolved as of early 2015.

Sources: References[7, 8]

Channel Cooperation

Cooperation by channel members is common in pharmacy. Cooperation often increases the efficiency and effectiveness of the overall channel so that all channel members benefit. Buying groups (or group purchasing organizations [GPOs]) are one example of channel cooperation in pharmacy. A buying group pools the purchasing power of a large number of individual pharmacies in order to negotiate better purchase prices from suppliers. The members of a buying group make an agreement to purchase all (or a high percentage) of selected items from contracted (or preferred) suppliers selected by the group. Those preferred suppliers give price discounts to group members in exchange for a steadier and more predictable revenue stream. Because of the volume of sales involved, the contracted suppliers are much more willing to provide lower prices to members of the buying group than to individual pharmacies.

Major pharmaceutical manufacturers often partner with pharmacists to help patients take their medicines as directed. They have funded pilot programs and research studies in the areas of medication therapy management and medication adherence. Funding these programs can provide a win-win-win solution where patients, pharmacies, and pharmaceutical companies all benefit. Patients get better health outcomes from appropriate medication use, and pharmacies and pharmaceutical companies increase sales of needed medications.

Members can be partners, allies, or competitors depending on the channel functions they choose to serve and whether other channel members compete for or cooperate in those functions. Roles within channels can change quickly depending on market conditions and strategic directions of partners. Table 3.2 shows potential functional roles of major channel members and potential opportunities for collaboration or conflict.

Table 3.2 Potential Functional Roles of Major Pharmaceutical Channel Members

CHANNEL MEMBERS

CHANNEL FUNCTION	Pharmacy / Pharmacist	Physician / Prescriber	PBM	Wholesaler	Insurance Plan	Patient
Production & Adding Value	X	X	X	X		X
Promotional Communications	X		X	X		
Distribution	X		X	X		
Storage	X			X		X
Financing & Payment	X		X	X	X	X
Risk Sharing	X	X	X	X	X	X
Regulation	X	X	X	X	X	X
Relationship Management	X	X	X	X	X	X

MANAGING CHANNEL CONFLICT

Conflict within pharmaceutical marketing channels is inevitable, but it can be managed. The first step is to understand your position of power within a channel. If your channel partner needs you more than you need them, you have greater power. Alternatively, if your partner has other equally good options to working with you, they have more power in the relationship. For example, if Walmart makes up 100% of the sales of a small supplier of a generic brand of herbal medicines, Walmart may have more power because the supplier can lose all of its business if Walmart severs the relationship. Therefore, the supplier will need to accommodate any demands made by Walmart. On the other hand, if the supplier offers a highly sought-after herbal brand of medicines that Walmart really wants, the supplier will have more power to negotiate with Walmart.

The level of power in a relationship impacts each partner's commitment to the other. If partners feel that they mutually benefit from working together more than with others, the commitment and channel relationship will be strong. Commitment to a relationship is a function of:[9]

o *The benefits of being in that relationship.* Businesses maintain relationships with channel partners who can help them in some way. In many cases, this involves helping partners make or save money in some way. Pharmacists who can develop a strong business case that they make or save more money for partners than competing partners will earn greater commitment from partners.

o *The costs of terminating that relationship.* Often, the cost of terminating a relationship keeps partners together. For instance, many pharmacists stay in dissatisfying relationships with PBMs, not because of the benefits received, but of the fear of lost access to PBM customers.[10]

o *Shared goals and values.* When partners share similar goals and values, they are likely to be committed to a partnership. Shared goals and values help partners better predict and understand each other's motives. When individuals have similar motivations and perceptions of the world, they are less likely to attribute negative causes to the actions of partners. For instance, channel partners that both share a patient-centered mindset are less likely to attribute negative motives to actions that help the patient but hurt a partner.

o *Trust.* More than any other factor associated with strong relationships, trust is necessary for the highest levels of commitment between partners.[9] Trust describes confidence in a relationship partner's reliability and integrity. It refers to questions such as: (1) Can my partner be relied upon to keep promises? (2) Does my partner act in a consistent, reliable manner? (3) Will my partner let me down when given a chance? (4) Does my partner care about my success? If a partner cannot be expected to act in a consistent, predictable manner and with integrity and honor, commitment will be difficult.

Managing commitment in channels requires pharmacists to effectively manage how partners perceive them and their contributions to the relationship. They must make a continual case for the value they provide to partners and the customers served by partners. They should seek partners who share similar goals and values and continually work to gain and maintain their partners' trust. When pharmacists lose the trust of partners, they should try to find ways of repairing that trust or look for other partners.

OMNI-CHANNEL RETAILING

Brian Jennings visited his local Walgreens to refill his prescription for Norvasc (amlodipine). He had his physician electronically send his prescription to his local Walgreens. Before going to the store, he searched online for the lowest price provider of his Norvasc and verified that Walgreens was the low cost provider near his house. While at the pharmacy, Brandon noticed an electronic shelf label for Neutrogena Men® Skincare lotion, a product that he had seen discussed in a blog post. To investigate what others had to say about the lotion, he scanned the barcode with the RedLaser app on his smartphone. Satisfied with the posted recommendations, he took a bottle off of the shelf and continued to the pharmacy department.

This example illustrates how shopping at pharmacies has changed in recent years. Technology advances have blurred the boundaries between physical and online retail pharmacy. Customers are now able to interact with retailers any time and any place using technologies like smartphones and other devices. The physical world of pharmacy is merging with online experiences via omnichannel retailing. Pharmacists will need to compete in an omnichannel environment to survive in the future.

Omnichannel retailing is defined as "an integrated sales experience that melds the advantages of physical stores with the information-rich experience of online shopping (Figure 3.5)."[11] Omni-channel has evolved from *multi-channel retailing* which refers to serving consumers with assorted channels like store, internet, and mail order but in a non-integrated way.

Omnichannel retailing tries to provide a seamless experience in which consumers switch back and forth through all available shopping channels. The omnichannel approach uses advanced customer relationship management (CRM) software to track consumers' experiences across all channels. Information collected from customer data, visits to store websites, loyalty programs, and participation in social networks is used to understand individual consumer preferences and habits. This allows retailers to better serve the needs of today's customer.

A digitally-adept customer who enters a brick-and-mortar pharmacy may have already searched for information about medications and expects pharmacy employees to know more than they do. This knowledge might extend beyond the drug to management of disease, health prevention recommendations, pricing, and what is best for that specific patient. In this environment, the pharmacist needs to know as much as possible about potential customers. With a few clicks of an electronic device, the pharmacist can access medication records, purchase history, preferred channels, and a range of other information. Solutions can be individualized for each patient using a mix of physical and online solutions working from the same Customer Relationship Management (CRM) database of information about patients.

Walgreens, CVS, and other major pharmacy chains have embraced omnichannel retailing. Walgreens engages with customers through Walgreens.com, Drugstore.com, and Beauty.com; mobile site visits, social media platforms, and the traditional brick-and-mortar store. When customers shop both the stores and online, they spend 3.5 times the average of a store-only customer.[12] When they engage with Walgreens across store, mobile, and web they spend six times as much as store-only customers.[12] In omnichannel retailing, the brick-and-mortar pharmacy becomes one option, albeit an important one, within the customer experience.

Figure 3.5 Omni-Channel Experience for the Pharmacy Customer

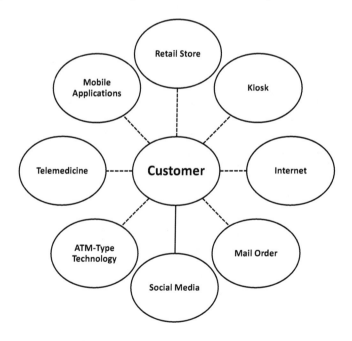

MARKETING IN ACTION

Popular Pharmacy Apps

Mobile pharmacy apps are new channels for serving customers. Almost all pharmacy chains and many independently owned pharmacies offer mobile apps to customers which provide a range of functions and tasks to be completed on smart phones. The most popular apps allow patients to:

- o transfer their prescriptions
- o compare prices
- o look up drug names and drug information
- o scan prescription vials for refills
- o receive coupons and offers
- o find the nearest pharmacy
- o rate and see ratings of pharmacies
- o remind them to take their medications
- o manage family prescriptions
- o go on virtual shopping trips
- o receive text messages
- o identify pills
- o check for drug interactions
- o manage insurance information
- o maintaining vaccination schedules

Apps are designed to facilitate the service experience for pharmacy customers. Typically, they increase customer control over their experiences by allowing them to complete routine tasks with a few key strokes of their smart devices. They can also improve communications with customers by reminding them about needs for vaccinations or texting them with information relevant to their care.

CONCLUSION

Roles of pharmacists in channels continue to change. Serving pharmacy customers requires collaboration with channel partners but often leads to conflict too. Pharmacists are intermediaries in most pharmacy channels, meaning that their value results from how well they serve their new and established roles within the supply chain. Pharmacists can add value in more ways than just by selling merchandise, and increasingly they are stepping into roles outside of the distribution function.

Opportunities can be found from moving from a product-dominant to a service-dominant logic to providing pharmacist services. This framework is consistent with trends in business and health care and allows pharmacists to move to a service-centric model of pharmacist care.

Reference List

(1) Wohlson M. How Robots and Military-Grade Algorithms Made Same-Day Delivery Possible. Wired.. 3-19-2013.

(2) Sherman L. E-Commerce: Three Ways Same-Day Delivery Will Change Retail. AdAge . 3-6-2013.

(3) Cavalla D. The extended pharmaceutical enterprise. Drug Discov Today 2003;8(6):267-274.

(4) Johnson SR. CVS decision to quit tobacco highlights its growing role as healthcare provider. Mod Healthc 2014;44(6):11.

(5) Kotler P, Shalowitz J, Stevens RJ. Strategic Marketing for Health Care Organizations. San Francisco, CA: Jossey-Bass; 2008.

(6) Kennelty KA, Chewning B, Wise M, Kind A, Roberts T, Kreling D. Barriers and facilitators of medication reconciliation processes for recently discharged patients from community pharmacists' perspectives. Res Social Adm Pharm 2014.

(7) Martin TW, Kell J. Walgreen, Express Scripts Sign Network Agreement. Wall Street Journal 2012 Jul 12.

(8) Silverman E, Ziobro P. CVS Plays Hardball With Rival Drug Chains. Wall Street Journal 2014 Oct 20.

(9) Morgan RM, Hunt SD. The commitment-trust theory of relationship marketing. the journal of marketing 1994;20-38.

(10) Talsma J. The PBM squeeze: Despite acute margin pressure, retail pharmacies fight to stay in the game. Drug Topics [April 15]. 4-15-2013.

(11) Rigby D. The future of shopping. Harvard Business Review 2011;89(12):65-76.

(12) Swerdlow F. The Walgreens Path to Omnichannel Success. 2-5-2013. National Retail Federation. 1-26-2015.

Exercises

1. Identify channels other than medication distribution in which pharmacist participate. Describe their roles in these channels.

2. Discuss how might the day-to-day routine of pharmacists change with next-hour shopping? What impact would this have on a pharmacist's role within the pharmacy?

3. Go to a general practice pharmacy publication like the Journal of the American Pharmacists Association and identify articles that deal directly or indirectly with channel conflict. Identify the channel members in the conflict and the source of the conflict. Which channel member has the most power in the conflict? Which channel member makes the best argument for serving patients or the general public?

4. Identify examples of channel cooperation between pharmacists and other intermediaries. Describe their areas of common interest and conflict. Discuss whether this cooperation is likely to be long-lasting.

PART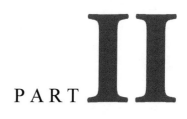

Marketing Strategy

CHAPTER 4

STRATEGIC PLANNING PROCESS

Co-authored by Norman Carroll

This chapter discusses the process of strategic planning for pharmacists. It describes how pharmacists can identify what they want to do and take steps to achieve it.

MARKETING IN ACTION

Yikes! What Will I Do?

Karen Wesley is a newly hired pharmacist who has been asked to plan and implement a diabetes clinic at an independent pharmacy. The pharmacy provides a broad range of merchandise, including complementary medicines, gourmet and international foods, and specialty gifts, for an upscale clientele. Clinical pharmacy services are a new and expanding offering for the independent.

In 2 weeks, Karen will be expected to present a marketing plan to the owner that delineates the program design, clientele served, local competition, and promotional strategy.

Karen wonders where to start.

SETTING ORGANIZATIONAL STRATEGIES

Mission

Most pharmacists work in health systems, pharmacy chains, governmental agencies, and other types of organizations. Each of these organizations is involved in business, meaning that they seek to achieve specific aims and purposes. Each has a mission which defines its core business, purpose, and reason for existence. An organization's mission may be explicitly stated or implied by how they conduct business. Explicit statements of an organization's mission are called mission statements.

A mission statement is a broad yet specific statement of an organization's purpose for existence and its future direction. The mission statement plays a critical role in strategic planning. All planning and strategies for future action originate (or should) from the mission of the organization

Most pharmacy organizations have a formal mission statement that describes the customers served, the needs the pharmacy fulfills for the customers, and the products and services provided to meet those needs. The mission (vision) statements for the three biggest pharmacy chains are presented below (accessed from company websites on 2/7/2015).

Rite Aid: To improve the health and wellness of our communities through engaging experiences that provide our customers with the best products, services and advice to meet their unique needs

Walgreens: To be America's most loved pharmacy-led health, wellbeing and beauty enterprise

CVS Health: We're a pharmacy innovation company and every day we're working to make health care better

Mission statements drive planning and decision-making. For instance, any initiative of Rite Aid should be consistent with offering "the best products, services and advice" in the form of an "engaging experience" which leads to "health and wellness of our communities." Any initiatives or practices inconsistent with the company mission can send mixed messages about the company and possibly damage public trust.

STRATEGIC TERMINOLOGY

The terms associated with strategies are often confused. Goals, strategies, objectives, and tactics guide how businesses achieve their missions. Understanding the differences is important.

Goals are broadly defined outcomes associated with the business mission. An example is "to be the number one pharmacy in the metropolitan area."

Strategies are the general approach used to achieve goals such as, "We will be the low cost leader in prescription medicines in the metropolitan area."

Objectives are specific measurable outcomes that are to be achieved within a designated time frame; "Our medication prices will be consistently the lowest in yearly surveys of prescription medications". To be useful in decision-making, objectives must be SMART.

o   **S**pecific – target a specific area for improvement

o   **M**easurable – quantify or at least suggest an indicator of progress

o   **A**ssignable – can specify who will do it

o   **R**ealistic – state what results can realistically be achieved, given available resources

o   **T**ime-related – specify when the result(s) can be achieved

An objective like "work harder and faster" is not SMART. A better objective might be to "the pharmacy department will increase the number of patients enrolled in our MTM program by 10% by the end of the year."

Tactics are the tools used in achieving the objectives associated with a strategy like "We will use robot dispensing technology to reduce the average cost of prescriptions filled in our pharmacy."

Strategy

A strategy is a plan for accomplishing goals and objectives. Strategic planning requires firms to develop a clear understanding of their present circumstances, identify where they want to be, and map a plan for getting there. It describes tactics to persuade customers to do business with you rather than your competitors. To achieve that, strategy must advance a unique combination of price, product, place, and promotion that gives you a competitive advantage in your market.

In most organizations, strategy comes from the top management. The chief executive in a typical pharmacy organization works with others in leadership positions to set a strategic direction for the organization. In a large pharmacy chain, the chief executive officer consults with other top executives on strategies. In an independent pharmacy, the pharmacist owner consults with managers and key employees.

The extent of pharmacists' involvement in developing organizational strategies depends on their job responsibilities, the business they work for, and their desire to become involved in the business. Strategic planning is a key responsibility in some pharmacist positions; this is more likely as pharmacists rise further within an organization. In some pharmacy organizations, everyone is encouraged to be involved in strategic planning, including staff pharmacists and technicians. This is most common in businesses that use an empowerment approach to management, in which many managerial decisions are delegated to employees who are encouraged to take responsibility for new business ideas. In such organizations, the only limitation to pharmacist participation in strategic planning is pharmacists' willingness to participate. Pharmacists who want to change pharmacy practice must be part of the strategic planning process.

Strategic planning occurs at various levels in large health care organizations: corporate, division, strategic business unit (SBU), and product.[1] For example, CVSHealth Corporation consists of retail, pharmacy benefit manager, retail medical clinic, and specialty medicine divisions. Senior management conducts strategic planning to coordinate the activities of these divisions. Under each of those divisions are SBU's which manage components of each division.[1] The makeup of a SBU will vary depending on the specific business. For example, SBUs in the retail division of pharmacy chain might be all pharmacies located within defined geographic areas, or within functions of the retail business like pharmacy, upfront merchandise, and online services.

Within each SBU are products (i.e., merchandise and services) which may have specific strategic plans. For example, an individual pharmacy within a chain might pilot a new medication reconciliation service associated with a local health system. It is at this product level that most pharmacist involvement occurs in the strategic planning process. Pharmacists may be involved in numerous local planning initiatives including implementation of MTM services, community based public health programs, and services targeted to a local long term care facility.

The main point for pharmacists to understand is that planning across the corporation, divisions, SBUs, and products must be coordinated and complimentary. Pharmacists who innovate within a large corporation must do so in a manner consistent with the company's mission and overall strategy. This means that initiatives at individual pharmacies must be in harmony with the store's SBU, division, and corporate strategy. One reason that the CVS pharmacy division and individual stores within the division stopped selling tobacco products was because it was inconsistent with CVSHealth Corporation's strategy to rebrand itself as a health care company.[2]

BUSINESS MODEL

A business model describes how a business or element of a business plans to make money. Business models are general, large picture views of the business and typically gloss over the operational details of the business. Clayton Christensen, known for coining the term "disruptive innovation", states that all business models boil down to three generic types:

Solution Shops: Solution shops are businesses that provide solutions for complicated problems that have few, if any, clear solutions. Any work done by experts who draw upon deep experience, training, and skills to serve customer's needs is done in solution shops. Solution shops typically get paid more for their services because they solve the hard problems that others cannot. Pharmacy examples include consulting firms, research & development organizations, some compounding pharmacies, and other businesses that provide highly customized solutions to clients.

Value-Adding Process Businesses: These businesses are typically intermediaries in marketing channels which take something from one channel partner (e.g., manufacturer), add value (e.g., repackage medications and provide counseling on proper usage), and then ship them out to the consumer or next intermediary. Any health care that can be guided by rules-based and standardized processes are value adding activities. This comprises most health care activities associated with primary care, surgical procedures, and routine diagnoses. The majority of pharmacies are value adding process businesses, because the problems they solve for patients are relatively routine and lend themselves to standardized treatment plans. This includes community, specialty, hospital, and managed care pharmacy services.

Facilitated Networks: Facilitated networks provide value by connecting people together via a platform through which users can offer things of value to each other. Facebook, YouTube, and other social media platforms are facilitated networks. Facilitated networks in pharmacy include pharmacy associations, pharmaceutical purchasing groups, some health insurance companies, and job search platforms. They provide value by connecting individuals and organizations. In most situations, more connections mean greater value. For example, the larger the pharmaceutical purchasing group, the more power group members have to negotiate lower prices from suppliers.

Business models contain at least three primary components.[3]

1. *Customer value proposition (CVP)*: A CVP is a description of how a business creates value for customers—by solving important problems better than anyone else. It is the case made for its utility to customers.

2. *Resources and processes*: Resources refer to the people, technology, merchandise, facilities, location, and other things needed to deliver the value proposition to the targeted customer. Processes describe the ways that operations and management use resources to deliver value in a sustainable way. These processes might include tasks like inventory control, purchasing, budgeting, information management, service design, and service management.

3. *Profit formula*: The profit formula defines how sufficient revenues are generated by the business to cover the costs of providing the CVP over time.

All business models attempt to describe how these three interdependent components result in a sustainable way of serving customers. To be sustainable, a business must be able to generate sufficient profits to maintain or support itself over the long term.

Community pharmacies often work under retail business models (RBM). Traditional RBMs generate the majority of their revenue by selling merchandise.[4] The problem with traditional RBMs is that few are unique. This makes them into commodities (i.e., undifferentiated and interchangeable). Many retail businesses, including community pharmacies, are now trying to move toward new RBMs that innovate with differentiated services and focus on enhancing customer experiences. This can be done by offering one of four primary customer value propositions: economic, functional, emotional, and symbolic.[4]

1. A business makes an *economic value proposition* when it argues that the marginal benefits (i.e., utility) it offers customers (compared to competitors) is greater than the costs and sacrifices paid.
2. A *functional value proposition* offers convenience by finding the right products with as little time and as little physical and cognitive effort as possible.
3. An *emotional value proposition* offers an arousal of feelings associated with the act of shopping itself, e.g., enjoying shopping with others, the hunt-for-a-bargain, relaxation.
4. Finally, a *symbolic value proposition* attaches positive consumption meanings associated with shopping itself e.g., shopping local, shopping that supports environment.

Pharmacy business models tend to rely on economic and functional arguments. Look at the marketing messages coming from most retail pharmacies. Most emphasize economic value propositions by promoting savings with coupons, rewards cards, sales, and other tactics. These are combined with functional value propositions which highlight fast service, mail order, drive thru, apps for mobile devices, 24-hour access, online services, one-stop-shopping, and other ways of getting what people need with minimal effort.

BUSINESS MODEL CANVAS

There are a variety of tools for planning and developing business models. One popular tool is the Business Model Canvas.[5] It is a template describing existing or creating new business models. It employs a visual chart to illustrate a firm's value proposition, targeted customers, revenue, costs, and other relevant model elements. An adapted business model canvas is shown in Figure 4-1.

Figure 4-1 Business Model Canvas for Pharmacy Services

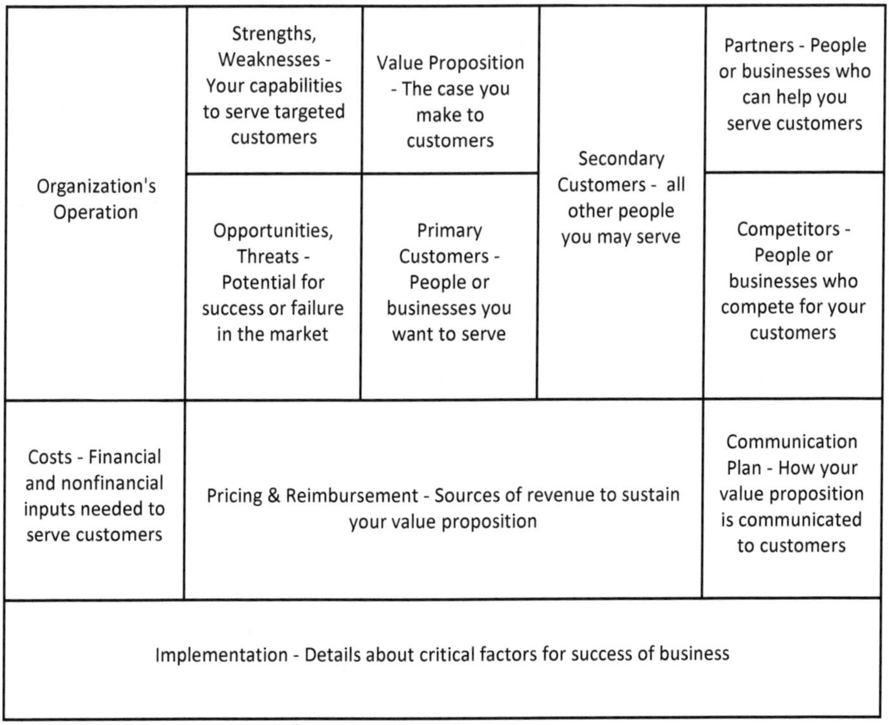

Organization's Operation	Strengths, Weaknesses - Your capabilities to serve targeted customers	Value Proposition - The case you make to customers	Secondary Customers - all other people you may serve	Partners - People or businesses who can help you serve customers
	Opportunities, Threats - Potential for success or failure in the market	Primary Customers - People or businesses you want to serve		Competitors - People or businesses who compete for your customers
Costs - Financial and nonfinancial inputs needed to serve customers	Pricing & Reimbursement - Sources of revenue to sustain your value proposition			Communication Plan - How your value proposition is communicated to customers
Implementation - Details about critical factors for success of business				

Source: Business Model Canvas (adapted) [5]

The value of the Business Model Canvas is its simplicity is in visually laying all of the major elements of the business plan onto one page. This helps in communicating the plan to others and in brainstorming sessions about plan details. Individuals involved in developing the model typically communicate their ideas by placing post-it notes directly on the canvas - continually adding, moving, and subtracting ideas in an iterative process.

By necessity and design, the Canvas only contains rough details about plans in order to adapt the plan as the business model evolves. Ideas on the canvas are only considered to be hypotheses that need to be tested by researching the market and interviewing people. This leads to continual revisions of the model as things are learned.

The business model canvas is often promoted for use in startup companies and for designing innovations,[5] although it can be used to develop outlines prior to writing detailed business plans. Further information about the Business Model Canvas and how to build them can be found on numerous websites including businessmodelgeneration.com and steveblank.com.

BUSINESS PLAN

A business plan is essentially a more detailed version of a business model. The business model describes how a business plans to thrive and the business plan lays out the steps for implementing the business model. In many cases, it is useful to flesh out the details of a business model before starting on the business plan.

The business plan is a blueprint on which all company decisions are based. The business plan contains goals and objectives for the operations of the organization. From those goals and objectives, strategies are formulated for finance, human resources, research and development, production, and marketing.

No Business Plan Survives First Contact With A Customer

Steve Blank, entrepreneur

Business plans are meant to evolve over time as one learns what works and does not work. Pharmacists should think of business plans as a process more than a document. Most elements of business plans are simply guesses about which customers to target or how they will respond to a marketing mix. Marketing messaging, pricing, service delivery, and other strategies typically change when they are used on real customers in real life settings. Successful pharmacists adapt as they learn.

Similar to business models, the business planning can concisely summarized by the following steps:

- ○ Analyze the market for opportunities and threats,
- ○ Assess the fit of one's mission, resources, and capabilities to the market environment,
- ○ Choose a course of action based on these analyses, and
- ○ Assess the success of the plan.

These steps may appear to be common sense, but pharmacists are typically not very good at business planning. Studies indicate that many pharmacy owners and managers do not conduct strategic planning, have little knowledge of the process, or do not consider it a priority in their practice.[6, 7] Like most people, pharmacists prefer action to planning. It can be difficult for pharmacists to take time for systematic planning when the immediate course of action seems obvious.

Many pharmacists start important marketing initiatives with only a vague idea of what they want to do. They may say, "Let's provide pharmaceutical care to our patients. We can develop brochures to give to patients and charge $1 for each minute spent with the patient. Let's get started."

In businesses of all types, starting a new service with only a sketchy plan is not uncommon. However, such a plan often dooms the new service to failure, because it does not consider the many issues and problems involved in the success of a new idea.

Business planning is difficult to be done successfully in one's head. It is useful to compile a written plan. Writing the plan helps focus ideas and ensures that important issues are not overlooked or ignored. A written plan prevents muddled thinking and makes it easier to share the plan with others.

The real value of the plan is not the plan itself, however. The value lies in the process of thinking through what you plan to do. As President Dwight Eisenhower eloquently put it, "Plans are worthless, but planning is everything."

MAJOR ELEMENTS OF A BUSINESS PLAN FOR PHARMACIST SERVICES

Details about business plans vary depending on how they are to be used. A plan submitted by an independent pharmacy to a bank for financing a new clinical service will differ from a major pharmacy chain's plan to enter a new market. The format and level of detail will vary depending on the intended audience, but there are some generally accepted elements expected in comprehensive business plans. This section describes what might be expected in a business plan for a new clinical service.

The Executive Summary. The Executive Summary provides an introduction to the plan and explains the major points of the plan "in a nutshell." Few people will spend the time to read an entire plan, so the Summary should be able to stand on its own without explanation. It often summarizes the following points:

- A brief description of the product or service that you plan to market

- A description of the purpose of the product or service, the individuals involved in its implementation (e.g., training, personal traits) and the organization where service will be provided (e.g., Medicine Shoppe, MCV outpatient clinic, CVS)

- A description of the value provided by the product or service

- A brief statement of the main marketing objectives and strategies contained in the plan including key assumptions with the plan, the target market, and positioning strategies

- Major financial details including revenues, start-up costs, operating costs, and break-even point

Product or Service Description. This section provides details about products and services being marketed and their competitive advantages. The description includes main features, channels through which the service/product will be delivered, the value proposition being made, and any other crucial details about what needs to be done to deliver on the value proposition and achieve success (e.g., a collaborative practice agreement with local physicians).

The Pharmacy's Operation. Specific background is given about the organization where the product/service will be provided. The descriptive information might include the organization's name, type of business, its mission, how it positions itself in the community (i.e., its positioning statement), and its portfolio of services and products. If not detailed elsewhere, this section may also provide specific information about key personnel.

SWOT Analysis. This section delineates the strengths and weaknesses of the pharmacy organization and the opportunities and threats in the market environment. The purpose is to identify important details about the organization or market environment that might influence the success of the product or service. Greater details about the SWOT analysis are provided later in this chapter.

Customers. Customers include all of the groups of individuals the product or service is expected to serve. This might include patients, family members, payers like insurance companies or employers, or physician practices. This section describes what problems will be solved by the proposed product/service for customers.

Primary Targeted Segments/Markets. This is a description of the primary target market of the business plan. It is a description of the segment or segments to be served, how they will be identified and targeted with promotional communications and offerings, and an estimate of the number of potential customers available to be served.

Partners. Partners are individuals or groups inside or outside of the pharmacy organization who may support the business plan in some way. These stakeholders have some interest in the plan and their participation or backing can benefit it in some way. Partners inside a chain pharmacy might be technicians, clerks, the store manager, other pharmacists (within the store and at other stores if in a chain), the district manager, information technology staff, and individuals in the corporate office. Partners outside of the organization could be physicians, local clinics & hospitals, other pharmacies in the area, employers, insurers, government, local pharmacy schools, professional associations, independent pharmacy groups (e.g., Good Neighbor), wholesalers, community organizations, and others.

Competitors. This describes primary competitors of the business. It might include direct (i.e., intra type) competitors like local pharmacies or pharmacy oriented businesses and indirect (i.e., intertype) competitors that meet similar customer needs and wants of targeted customers.

Revenue, Pricing, and Costs. Relevant financial details are provided like costs, pricing, and revenues of the business. It explains how the business will receive revenue for the service or product being provided--direct payment or indirect financial benefits coming through cost savings, increased upfront sales, or other benefits. It also describes the costs of providing the service and how pricing will generate sufficient revenue to cover the costs. This is typically explained in financial statements of forecasted or estimated yearly sales, estimated net income, and break-even points.

Promotional Plan. Promotional objectives and communication strategies are discussed for positioning the service or product to convey a distinct, desired image to customers. This section explains messaging (e.g., personalized, professional care) and delivery strategies (e.g., point-of-sale signage, personal selling). It should explain the unique selling proposition used, describe the communication mix, and the discuss communications budget details.

Implementation Plan. This section discusses the most important things needed to successfully implement the program. This might include new software, changes in workflow, shifting greater responsibilities to the technicians, and remodeling the pharmacy. It might mention what customers must do for the program to succeed (e.g., Do patients need to learn new behaviors or be able to access certain technologies like a mobile phone or Internet?). Finally, it should discuss performance measures that indicate the success of the plan such as the number of customers needed to be served.

MARKETING IN ACTION

Positioning Pharmacist Services

Positioning describes how marketers attempt to communicate *a desired, distinct image to customers*. It tries to develop a marketing mix (Price, Place, Promotion, and Product) that provides a consistent and powerful image of pharmacists and their business. Promotion is a major component of any positioning strategy; however, price, place, and product are also a part of positioning.

It is vital that a pharmacist's marketing mix be clear, distinct, and valued in the mind of customers. This sentence bears repeating. IT IS VITAL THAT A PHARMACIST'S MARKETING MIX BE CLEAR, DISTINCT, AND VALUED IN THE MIND OF CUSTOMERS.

If customers do not perceive a clear benefit, then pharmacists have no advantage over competitors. Businesses that do a poor job of differentiating themselves in the minds of customers become commodities.

A commodity is a product category that has no unique characteristics valued by customers. When consumers cannot perceive any differences between products in a market, those products become a commodity. To most people, gasoline is a commodity. The gasoline at one gas station is considered as good as the gas at any other station, so quality is not an issue. As with most commodities, people tend to rely on price and location in selecting gas stations. This example should cause some discomfort among pharmacists, since price and location are often cited as the primary reasons for selecting pharmacies. If price and location ever become the only reasons for selection, it will mean that pharmacies and pharmacists have not achieved a distinct perception of value in the minds of their patients—that they have become commodities. At that moment, pharmacists will have lost the marketing battle.

Successful positioning strategies use a marketing mix that is difficult to imitate. Although it may be easy for a competitor to imitate a pharmacist's patient education leaflets or brochures, it is difficult for a competitor to duplicate the interactions that excellent pharmacists have with patients. The trust and friendships developed by pharmacists who are close to their customers cannot be easily copied. Individual pharmacists often provide a competitive advantage for their pharmacy.

The overarching goal of positioning is to give patients a reason to choose your services over your competitors. This can be accomplished by identifying and highlighting key advantages that pharmacists have over their competition. By offering patients just one or two clear benefits, pharmacists can establish and maintain a competitive advantage.

SWOT ANALYSIS

One of the first steps of any business plan is an analysis of the strengths (S) and weaknesses (W) of the marketing organization, followed by an evaluation of opportunities (O) and threats (T) in the market.

Information from this SWOT analysis is used to develop and implement the rest of the business plan. The S and W of SWOT analysis are an assessment of the organization's resources—its strengths and weaknesses within the market. To survive in a market, an organization has to capitalize on its strengths and overcome its weaknesses. The O and T describe the analysis of the market environment and are intended to help understand the world in which the organization operates.

SWOT analyses are conducted to support major business decisions. A SWOT analysis might be conducted when an organization is deciding about the feasibility of a new service (e.g., diabetes management). The purpose is to discover any distinct advantage for a pharmacy in the current environment, upon which a strategy can be built. SWOT analysis might also be used to discover any weaknesses that make a pharmacy vulnerable to competitors or prevent it from succeeding.

A clear understanding of the competition is an important part of SWOT analysis. Capabilities and the market environment are assessed by comparing the company with competitors. If location is considered a strength, it is a strength in comparison with competitors. Similarly, price is considered in relation to competitors' prices.

There are no cookbook methods for SWOT analysis. No two SWOT analyses are alike. Each depends on the market, competition, and characteristics of the marketing organization.

Assessment of the Organization's Strengths and Weaknesses

This assessment attempts to clarify the current and potential capacity of an organization to compete in a market. It identifies strengths that give an organization an important advantage over competitors. These might include a well-known brand name, superior employees, strong company finances, or things the company is particularly good at doing. The capability assessment also identifies weaknesses that might hinder the company in the market. Weaknesses might include assets the company lacks or things the company does poorly in comparison with competitors. As much as possible, strengths and weaknesses should be assessed from the customer's point of view. A pharmacy may consider it a strength that all its pharmacists are residency trained, but if this is not important to customers, or if it doesn't result in service offerings that customers want then, it's not really a strength.

One way to conduct this assessment is to take a sheet of paper and list your organization's strengths and weaknesses. Try to think of every characteristic of the business. Then use another sheet to list the strengths and weaknesses of competitors. If you do not have enough information to do this, you need to visit your competitors. Assessing the capability of competitors should suggest strengths and weaknesses to add to your own list.

Not all attributes of a company are equally important, and the importance of each attribute to the overall success of the strategic business plan should be considered. Perceptions of price are likely to be more important to the success of a disease management program than promotional displays are. One way to assess importance is to determine which attributes of the business are most difficult to copy. A company that has superior employees and managers has important advantages that are not easily duplicated. When pharmacists think about strengths and weaknesses, they might consider answering the questions in Table 4-1.

Table 4-1 Questions to Answer in Identifying Strengths and Weaknesses

Strength or Weakness?	Questions to consider
Reputation	How loyal are patients to your pharmacy?
	How well does your reputation compare to your competitors?
	Do people recommend your pharmacy to others?
	What does social media (e.g., YELP) say about your pharmacy? How does it compare to other pharmacies?
	If your store is part of a chain or network, what is the reputation of your chain or network? How does it compare to other chains?
	What is your reputation with physicians and other health care providers in the area?
People	Do customers ask for your pharmacists and techs by name?
	What unique expertise do your people have (e.g., credentials)?
	Is management engaged and supportive of what you do?
	Does management provide effective leadership?
	Do employees and management have a marketing mindset?
	How committed are employees to the success of the organization?
Marketing	Do you have a particular advantage in the area when it comes to things like perceived price, convenience, location, promotional messaging, merchandise and service selection, unique products or services that cannot be found elsewhere, relationships with physicians and other health care providers in the area, or quality processes and procedures?
Resources	Are employees already working at capacity?
	Does the organization have the employee and management commitment needed to succeed in the marketplace?
	Does the organization have the money needed to succeed in the marketplace?
	Does the organization have the technology needed to support the product or service?
	How well does the layout of the pharmacy support efforts to serve patients?

Assessment of the Opportunities and Threats in the Market

This assessment is typically conducted in concert with strength and weakness assessment. They are considered together because the environment has a significant effect on the relative capabilities of organizations and competitors. An influx of immigrants or the opening of a new factory in a community might give some firms an advantage over others.

An opportunity analysis identifies gaps between market demand and what is currently available. It also analyzes potential changes in the market that may enhance the prospects for services or products. An opportunity analysis might ask:

- What needs are not being met in the current marketplace?

- How can our organization meet these needs better than competitors?

- How is the environment changing to the organization's advantage or disadvantage?

Opportunities can be found almost anywhere, if we keep our eyes open. One way of identifying opportunities is to continually scan the environment for new trends and changes. Opportunities can be found in discussions with customers, through reading magazines and newspapers and surfing the Internet, and by examining the trade literature.

Opportunities should be assessed for their desirability and their likelihood of success. Desirable opportunities are those most likely to generate a profit or make some contribution to the organization's mission. Likelihood of success is based on the capabilities of the organization, the capabilities of competitors, and the changing nature of the market.

A threat analysis attempts to identify unfavorable factors that might injure the business. Like opportunities, threats are identified by scanning the environment for relevant trends and market changes. An analysis of threats should consider the seriousness of the threat as well as the likelihood of its occurring. A threat analysis might ask:

- What potential problems might threaten the success of the organization's initiatives?

- What potential new competitors might arise? How might the organization's current competitors respond?

- What changes may be occurring in the environment to make our product or service obsolete?

- How might governmental policies, changing customer demographics, or a recession affect our organization's product or service?

- How might changes in customers' tastes affect demand?

o   What major trends will significantly affect our organization and the market?

Threat analysis identifies situations that can be influenced by marketing actions and those that cannot. With situations that can be influenced, such as the entry of a major competitor into the area, problems can be minimized or even turned into opportunities if sufficient time is available. For instance, major competitors can sometimes thrive side by side if they offer a different mix of services and products. For situations that cannot be influenced, new ways of adapting must be found.

MARKETING IN ACTION

Opportunities Associated with ACOs

Accountable Care Organizations (ACOs) are new healthcare entities that offer opportunities for pharmacists. Originating from the 2010 Affordable Care Act (ACA), ACOs have been encouraged as a way of coordinating care and improving chronic disease management. ACOs are groups of health care providers like hospitals, physician clinics, long-term care organizations, and pharmacies that work together in a formal ACO structure. ACOs are given financial incentives to achieve healthcare quality goals and save money.

Pharmacies can become part of ACOs because of their ability to influence:

o   Hospital readmissions. Pharmacists can help providers of Medicare services avoid lower reimbursement penalties levied for having high readmission rates within 30 days of a hospital discharge. Pharmacists can help reduce readmissions by improving medication adherence and improving transitions of care.

o   Patient experience and satisfaction. Hospital reimbursements may soon be affected by how patients rate their overall care experience. Community pharmacists will be a part of that experience and can affect satisfaction scores.

o   Partnerships. Many ACO's do not have the experience to effectively control pharmacy costs and outcomes. Pharmacists can contract with ACO's for medication therapy services and help ACOs meet contracted promises to improve quality of care and control costs.

Source: Reference[8]

IMPLEMENTING THE MARKETING PLAN

Even the best-conceived marketing plans can fail if they are poorly implemented. Successful implementation of marketing plans can be hindered in several ways. Sometimes poor implementation is just a failure to follow the plan. This can occur when not all people in the organization understand the plan and their roles. In other cases, implementation may suffer if people lose sight of the mission. In still other situations, structural limitations of the business can limit the success of some ideas. The following problems are often associated with implementation.

- o Insufficient commitment from management. When XYZ pharmacy decides to offer disease management services as part of its strategy, upper management of XYZ can hurt the implementation if it is not sufficiently committed to the idea. Lack of commitment may cause management to do things that make success difficult. Management may cut funding or staff. That is why it is so important to align clinical pharmacy initiatives with the mission and other business initiatives. If the new clinical service complements other things the business is doing, management will be more likely to support it.

- o Lack of staff commitment or expertise. Implementation can also fail because of insufficient commitment or expertise at the staff level. The best plan in the world will fail if people are unwilling or unable to follow it. A marketing plan that does not take into account the strengths and limitations of employees and managers in a company is likely to fail. For example, the implementation of medication therapy management services requires pharmacists who are competent, flexible, and enthusiastic about challenges. Not all pharmacists fit this description. Some are just not interested in stepping outside their traditional dispensing roles. Others may be uncomfortable with new tasks, or interested but not trained in providing higher levels of care. If such human limitations are not addressed, the marketing plan can fail.

- o Insufficient or bad information. Many marketing decisions are made with bad or insufficient information. Decisions are based on faulty assumptions about the business and the market. If managers assume that consumers care about only price and convenience, they will ignore the potential for patient care services. If managers lack information about competitors, customers, and the market, they will rely on past experience or assumptions that may not be relevant or appropriate to current conditions.

- o Structural contradictions. Marketing strategy often dictates a course of action that is inconsistent with the structural characteristics of the organization. Strategy may recommend that employees take greater responsibility in handling customers, while employee personnel policies inhibit or even punish employees who do so. Marketing strategies must be developed with explicit consideration of the structural characteristics of the organization. Successful implementation of marketing plans may require changes in structural aspects of the business, such as operating procedures and redesign of workflow and facilities.

o   Overextension. In most organizations, there are too many marketing tasks to accomplish with current resources and personnel. As a result, company leaders often try to do too many things and are unable to do any of them well. A pharmacy may wish to provide outstanding dispensing services, on-demand immunizations and clinical services, community outreach, and patient callbacks. Trying to do all of these things may result in failure of all of them. Successful implementation requires that choices be made.

REASSESSING

A feedback and control system should be put in place to evaluate the success of programs and identify ways in which they can be improved. Such a system could consist of a scheduled review of marketing programs and an action plan to address problems.

At the beginning of any program, a decision needs to be made about how to determine whether it is successful. This requires that measures of success or failure be collected. Measures of successful pharmacy services might consist of the total number of patients who use the service, revenue collected from the service, and patient satisfaction. The key is to identify the minimum number of easy-to-collect measures that can validly determine the success of the program.

When it is time to evaluate a program, a decision can be made to continue the program without changes, cancel the program, or make changes. Changes can include expansion of programs, contraction of programs, or adjustments designed to improve programs. In an ideal situation, a continuous quality improvement method should be used. Continuous quality improvement consists of applying the best methods from the literature to the pharmacy's own practice, using statistical quality improvement techniques to measure the results, and then using what was learned to make improvements. Pharmacists may choose instead to rely on their own personal judgment when reassessing efforts. A pharmacist who maintains close contact with the operations and patients of a pharmacy probably has a good idea of which strategies work and which do not, without the need for extensive statistical analyses.

SUMMARY

The ability to develop a strategic business plan is an important skill for pharmacists who wish to market their services. The steps to strategic business planning have been presented in a way that permits any pharmacist to write and implement a plan.

Marketing is not an event, but a process.... It has a beginning, a middle, but never an end, for it is a process. You improve it, perfect it, change it, even pause it. But you never stop it completely.

Jay Conrad Levinson, advocate of "guerrilla marketing"

Reference List

(1) Kotler P, Shalowitz J, Stevens RJ. Strategic Marketing for Health Care Organizations. San Francisco, CA: Jossey-Bass; 2008.
(2) Johnson SR. CVS decision to quit tobacco highlights its growing role as healthcare provider. Mod Healthc 2014;44(6):11.
(3) Christensen CM, Bohmer R, Kenagy J. Will disruptive innovations cure health care? Harv Bus Rev 2000;78(5):102-12, 199.
(4) Sorescu A, Frambach RT, Singh J, Rangaswamy A, Bridges C. Innovations in Retail Business Models. Journal of Retailing 2011;87, Supplement 1(0):S3-S16.
(5) Osterwalder A, Pigneur Y. Business Model Generation: A Handbook for Visionaries, Game Changers, and Challengers. Hoboken, NJ.: John Wiley and Sons; 2010.
(6) Harrison DL. Effect of attitudes and perceptions of independent community pharmacy owners/managers on the comprehensiveness of strategic planning. J Am Pharm Assoc (2003) 2006;46(4):459-464.
(7) Harrison DL, Ortmeier BG. Strategic planning in the community pharmacy. J Am Pharm Assoc (Wash) 1996;NS36(9):583-588.
(8) What ACOs Could Mean for Your Business. Smart Retailing . 5-28-2013.

Chapter Questions

1. Write a mission statement for a pharmacy where you would want to work.

2. How do medication therapy services or other clinical services fit into the overall business plan of your current or future pharmacy employer?

3. What is the purpose of a SWOT analysis? When should it be conducted? Why is knowledge of the competition important in a SWOT analysis?

4. Discuss opportunities and threats to the provision of medication therapy management in the average community pharmacy.

5. Describe common pharmacy practices that you believe enhance or hurt the image of pharmacists as health care professionals.

CHAPTER **5**

MARKETING STRATEGIES

Objectives

After studying this chapter, the reader should be able to

- o Contrast price from differentiation strategies
- o Identify how pharmacist service strategies might vary at different stages of the product life cycle
- o Discuss the principle of product portfolio management and how it might be used by pharmacists
- o Compare the benefits and potential downsides of convenience strategies used by pharmacies
- o Define the term shopper marketing and how it seeks to influence the customer's shopping experience
- o Suggest questions pharmacists can use to assess the ethics of their strategies

Pharmacists use many strategies to market pharmacist services and pharmacy products. This chapter focuses on the general business strategies used in pharmacy practice.

MARKETING IN ACTION

More, Better, Cheaper

A study in April 2014 found that many consumers would choose retail health clinics and other more affordable and convenient alternatives over traditional health care options.[1] Half of people surveyed preferred at-home or retail options to treat strep throat, administer chemotherapy, or receive other health care. The preference for non-traditional health care was greater for young people and individuals struggling with healthcare expenses. Patient cost-sharing is likely to increase this trend.

This means that within the next 10 years, health care may start to look more like consumer-oriented, technology-enabled industries such as Amazon and Google.[1] New companies will emerge to give consumers easy access to their personal health records, allow patients and health care providers to track health and healthcare, and offer other innovations at different prices and levels of intensity. Traditional health care businesses that cannot adapt will go out of business.

Pharmacies have jumped onto the trend toward consumer centered health care. For example, Walgreens offers a branded fitness tracker to more that 1 million of its customers.[2] The Walgreens Activity Tracker tracks sleep, distances traversed, and calories consumed. The tracker syncs with other Walgreens software like the Balance Rewards app which rewards users with points for completing healthy activities like recording weight and tracking blood pressure and glucose levels. The app also works with other fitness devices including Fitbit and iHealth.

Other Walgreens initiatives include an augmented reality app for in-store promotions, a mobile app that records customers' immunization history and recommendations for further immunizations, and a mobile app that allows users to consult online with a physician from their computer, tablet or phone. Not all of these apps are available nationwide yet.

Source: References [1] and [2]

GENERAL MARKETING STRATEGIES

There are many strategies to succeed in business, but they all boil down into two general strategies: be cheaper (i.e., the low cost option) or be different (i.e., differentiation strategy). All business strategies are some variation on these two approaches.

Low Cost Strategies

Cost-based strategies are used by businesses that attempt to be seen as the cheapest provider of merchandise or services. Businesses that use this strategy attempt to identify and exploit opportunities that reduce their costs below competitors'--primarily by being more efficient. Efficiency is increased by designing workplace environments that simplify and facilitate work, using systems that reduce wasted effort, targeting customers who are more profitable to the firm, motivating employees to work harder and smarter, and so on.

Businesses that are exceptional in lowering costs compete by being low cost leaders within their markets. Low cost leaders undercut the prices of competitors. If they offer the lowest prices, they can win customers away from competitors. Of course, lower prices mean lower profit margins, but the additional customers who are attracted to the low prices allow the business to remain profitable. To remain low cost leaders, they continually invest profits into developing new ways of doing business that further reduce cost.

Wal-Mart department stores are famous for their low-cost business strategy. Wal-Mart uses its tremendous purchasing power (i.e., thousands of stores) and efficient supply chain (i.e., own fleet of trucks, warehouses, and technology) to undercut prices of less efficient competitors. This forces competitors to react to Wal-Mart's prices and become price followers.

Low Cost Strategies in Health Care

Low cost strategies depend on how businesses define the market they want to serve. Pharmacies that see themselves as low cost providers of drugs will compete by offering the cheapest drugs to customers. They will buy drugs cheaply from manufacturers and wholesalers, keep service expenses at rock bottom levels by being frugal with salaries and staffing, and accept lower profit margins for invested capital. Pharmacies that define their market differently might use different low cost tactics.

The total costs in any health care market are a function of three variables in the following equation:

$$Cost = f(P,V,I)$$

P = Price of a service or product
V = Volume or amount of services or products provided (number of products or units of service)
I = Intensity of service (level of service e.g., nurse practitioner versus physician specialist)

The cost equation makes clear that there are a limited number of ways to lower health costs in the market for pharmaceuticals: (1) lower the price of drugs and/or services, (2) reduce the volume of drugs and/or services provided, (3) lower the intensity of care, or (4) offer a combination of the first three.

Each of these variables are interrelated (e.g., lowering price often increases sales, intense care often costs more), so influencing one or two without controlling for the others typically does not control overall costs. Instead, it simply shifts costs to other parts of the health care system (e.g., lowering the intensity pharmacist services may lead to additional emergency room visits and hospitalizations).

This suggests an alternative low cost strategy where pharmacists expand the market they serve to all of health care. Then pharmacists can make a case for lowering overall health care costs to institutional customers (i.e., health systems, accountable care organizations). In these conditions, the pharmacy low cost leader might be able to make a case for spending more on pharmacist services if it can be seen as driving down spending on other elements of health care like hospitalizations and emergency room visits.

Differentiation Strategies

Price becomes less important when businesses are seen by customers as offering a product or service package that is of higher quality, performs better, or is uniquely desirable. Businesses that differentiate themselves from competitors do so by offering a distinctive mix of products and services that are highlighted by effective advertising and promotion.

Differentiation strategies emphasize value more than price competition. Customers buy differentiated products and services because they perceive that they are getting more for their money. A desire for the lowest price is replaced by a desire for the highest value. Pharmacies often try to differentiate themselves from competitors by providing greater levels of service. This might mean faster, friendlier, more varied, or more convenient service.

Don't be afraid of being different. Be afraid
of being like everyone else.

- Anonymous

Niche Strategies

While some differentiation strategies target large customer populations,
other strategies identify narrow market segments (or niches) that have been
ignored, overlooked, or taken for granted by competitors. Many independent
pharmacies successfully compete with large chains by giving greater attention to
the local community. Focusing on narrow geographic niches, independent
pharmacists are often active in local organizations and more familiar with
neighborhood needs and interests than are employees of large chains. Their
closeness to the community can generate goodwill that gives them a competitive
advantage over larger firms.

This type of strategy focuses on the needs of a profitable few. Rather than
compete for all customers in a market, firms compete for a limited number of
profitable customers whom the firms can serve better than their competitors.
Pharmacists have attempted to serve the following niches: diabetes, asthma,
cholesterol, lab services, reproductive health, vaccines, hospice, AIDS, veterinary
services, smoking cessation, hypertension, complementary medicines,
anticoagulation services, postal delivery, and others.

SPECIFIC MARKETING STRATEGIES

PRODUCT LIFE-CYCLE STRATEGIES

The idea of product life cycles is that, like plants and animals, products have a
life. Each product life cycle has four stages: introduction, growth, maturity, and
decline. Sales volume and profitability vary over time as products progress
through each stage (Figure 5-1). By identifying a product's life-cycle stage, a
marketer can develop strategies with increased chances for success, including
health care.[3, 4]

Figure 5-1 Sales and profits within a product's life cycle

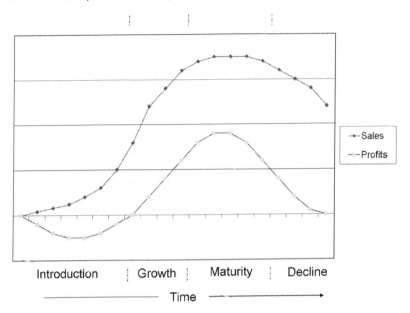

The product life-cycle concept permits a business to understand sales of a single product or group of products within a market. Life-cycle strategies are most commonly used for products that are exceptional, meet an unrealized need, and are unknown to the general market.

Introduction

New products or brands in the introduction stage are unique and face no immediate, direct competition. The goal of marketing is to introduce the product to consumers and induce them to try it. Since the product is new, sales growth is slow initially and profits are negative. The amount of money spent on promoting the product exceeds the revenue from sales. Promotional dollars are spent to educate consumers about the product's existence. Sales promotions, coupons, and price discounts attempt to persuade consumers to try the product. Money put into the product at this stage is an investment that the business hopes will pay off in later stages of the life cycle.

In community pharmacy practice, most clinical services are still in the introduction stage. These services fulfill a latent need, but they are often not profitable because they are not widely known or accepted. Significant money and effort still need to be expended before these services can move into the growth stage. Unless sufficient effort is spent promoting clinical services in community pharmacy, they risk dying a premature death.

Growth

In the growth stage, demand for the product starts to rise. Sales accelerate rapidly, climbing initially at an increasing pace and then at a decreasing rate toward the end of the growth stage. Since there are few competitors in the market at the beginning of the growth stage, high prices can be charged, and profits start to move into positive territory.

As the product moves through the growth stage, competitors start to enter the market to gain a share of the profits. This puts pressure on prices and profits. Early entrants into the market must either lower prices in response or offer innovations that justify higher prices. The first, innovative product on the market typically has an advantage over later market entrants, because significant experience and brand awareness can be gained in the introduction stage. This experience can be used to stay one step ahead of competitors.

Pharmacist administered vaccines are currently in a growth phase. Many community pharmacists are aggressively promoting influenza, shingles, and other vaccinations in their stores. As vaccination becomes widely available, competition will likely force pharmacists to lower their prices or compete with higher levels of service.

Maturity

In the maturity stage, sales reach their peak and start to decline. Profits begin to erode. This stage is typically the longest one; for some products it can last decades. Although profits erode in the maturity stage, they can still be sufficient. In this stage, the goal of marketers is to defend their share of the market from competitors. This can be done by constantly refining the marketing mix.

Dispensing services have been in the maturity stage for many years. They are unchanged in many respects from 50 years ago. Most competition in dispensing has been through minor improvements designed to attract different market segments, improve quality, and drive down prices. Innovations such as drive-through windows, Internet services, and telephone refill services have permitted pharmacies to prolong the maturity phase of dispensing services.

Decline

During this stage, sales and profits decrease until the product is withdrawn from the market. Like any living organism, a product reaches a stage where it can no longer survive. Consumer tastes may change, or a new competitor may dry up demand in the market. Whatever the reason, products eventually decline and disappear from the market. Manual typewriters and the slide rule eventually disappeared from the market, and this will happen to many services and products provided by pharmacists.

> Dream as if you'll live forever. Live as if you'll
> die today.
>
> - James Dean

Understanding product life cycles provide perspective for pharmacists who implement new programs. Any new idea, such as MTM, takes time and effort to bear fruit. During the introduction stage, time, effort, and patience on the part of the pharmacist are required. Pharmacists should not expect immediate payoff.

If an idea is successful enough to move into the desirable growth stage, a lot of work needs to be done to keep it there. As business explodes in the growth stage, demand may look as if it will never end. However, as competitors move into growing markets, it is more difficult to increase and sustain sales and profits. As an idea moves into the maturity stage, it takes constant marketing to keep it thriving. Finally, when the product is no longer profitable, it must be removed from the market.

PORTFOLIO STRATEGIES

A portfolio is all the products and services offered by a business. A portfolio strategy helps define the mix of products and services that a business offers. All community pharmacies practice some form of portfolio strategy whenever they make a choice to add or subtract products and services from their stores.[5, 6]

The purpose of a portfolio is to choose the right mix of products and services to meet the demand of customers as efficiently and effectively as possible. Figure 5-2 shows a way of displaying products in a portfolio matrix that helps identify which products and services to keep or delete.

Products within the matrix can be classified in various ways. In this matrix, products are classified by the extent to which they are profitable and increasingly generate sales revenue. For other businesses, matrix variables might be market share, impact on reputation, or some other important variable. Use of the matrix helps determine whether a product should receive greater investments, have its cash cow harvested for other parts of the business, or be dropped from the portfolio.

Figure 5-2 Portfolio Matrix

Profitability of this
Product or Service

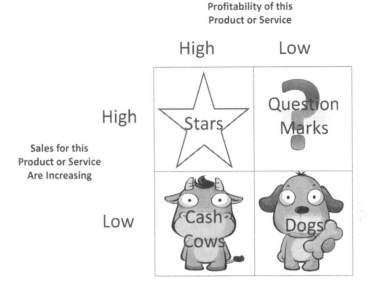

Within the matrix, "cash cows" are products that are typically valuable to the business but not growing in sales. In the matrix in Figure 5-2, cash cows are profitable, generating excess cash for a business, but not growing in sales or likely to grow in the future. The strategy with cash cows is to milk them for cash or whatever other value they can provide but to direct minimal resources to them. The idea is that since they are unlikely to grow with more effort, then resources should be put elsewhere. The strategy is to maintain the status quo.

"Stars" are profitable, growing in sales, and likely to offer potential for even greater future growth. Because of their potential, resources are invested in these products and services. As stars age, they eventually become cash cows. Right now, medication synchronization and immunization services are stars in many pharmacies. They are fast-growing markets and their potential justifies the money spent on promoting them and building their infrastructure.

"Question marks" are products that are not profitable and where the potential to increase sales is not clear. Typically, their performance is weak but might be improved with greater marketing efforts. Medication therapy management services can be classified as question marks in most community pharmacies. The potential benefit of MTM may be worth the cost but it will take time and effort to know.

"Dogs" are products that provide little value to the business and can be a drain on resources. Dogs are typically deleted from the portfolio.

To assess and fine tune a pharmacy service/product portfolio, pharmacists need to follow several steps.

1. Identify your primary target markets, such as patients with certain disease states, patients of particular physicians, certain age groups, or managed care customers.

2. Inventory your current service offerings. Most pharmacies provide basic dispensing services that are supported by front-end merchandise purchases. Other potential services might be counseling, disease management, screening for conditions such as osteoporosis, vaccinations, durable goods fittings, home health care, and nursing home services.

3. Identify which of your current services are viable in your target markets. The goal is to offer different levels of services depending on the target market. For instance, managed care companies may be open to proposals for certain disease management or vaccination programs that complement basic dispensing services. Seniors may be willing to pay for extensive counseling about their prescriptions.

4. Identify which services you need to add or subtract to round out your service portfolio. Selection depends on the value of each service to your various target markets and the cost of providing the service. Services can be assessed for their importance to customers, customer willingness to pay, and a service's overall contribution to the service portfolio.

The goal is to match the right services and products to the needs of target segments at the lowest costs. This means that each item in the portfolio must have a purpose. Cash Cows generate revenue that supports the potential of Stars and Question Marks. Stars and Question Marks are investments in the future of the pharmacy. Any items that no longer have a clear purpose in the portfolio can be labeled dogs and deleted from the portfolio.

An additional consideration in evaluating a product or service is how it might help balance the portfolio. Although some products do not generate much cash or have high growth potential, they can add balance to the overall portfolio. A cholesterol screening program might not generate much immediate revenue for the pharmacy or have much potential for doing so in the future. However, it can benefit the product and service portfolio of the pharmacy by complementing the other disease management offerings, generating store traffic, and enhancing the image of the pharmacy in the community.

CONVENIENCE STRATEGIES

A major way that pharmacies differentiate themselves is through convenience strategies.[7-11] Most community pharmacies have made convenience an important part of their overall marketing strategy where they try to offer greater speed and ease of shopping to pharmacy services and merchandise.

This makes sense, because research has consistently found location and convenience to be important factors in consumer patronage of pharmacies.[7-9] In fact, pharmacy uses convenience to differentiate itself from other professions, referring to the pharmacist as the "most accessible health care professional."

Convenience generally refers to speed and ease of shopping. This includes the ability to shop at one location, availability of store directories, clearly marked merchandise and prices, a good store layout, easy traffic flow in the aisles, minimal out-of-stock merchandise, no waiting in lines, omnichannel marketing, and expanded operating hours.

But convenience means different things to different people. For parents with small children, it might mean having prescriptions filled without getting out of the car. For a housebound disabled person, it might mean being able to shop from home. For a young, healthy shopper, it might mean easy parking and one-stop shopping for clothing, groceries, household goods, and drugs.

The push for customer convenience has been responsible for many changes in the practice of pharmacy. Convenience is the reason pharmacies are located in supermarkets, shopping malls, and mass merchandisers (e.g., Target, Kmart, and Wal-Mart). It is the reason for drive-through, mail order, and Internet pharmacies.

The Downside of Convenience Strategies

One problem with convenience strategies is that the demand for greater convenience never ends. Each time a pharmacy offers a convenience innovation, consumers quickly become accustomed to it and expect further improvement. Moreover, the advantage of a convenience improvement fades when competitors copy it. Also, innovations of non-pharmacy businesses raise consumer expectations of convenience. When consumers see that a bank transaction worth thousands of dollars can be completed in 30 seconds, they begin to wonder why a prescription can't be filled in the same amount of time.

> Every convenience brings its own
> inconveniences along with it.
>
> -Anonymous

Pharmacy services that are now considered convenient will be regarded as slow in the future. Consider photo processing. Consumers used to wait days or weeks to have photographs developed and returned to them. Pharmacies started offering 24-hour photo processing, then 1-hour processing, but some consumers soon found these services too slow. Now, photo processing on demand competes with digital cameras that share photos in the virtual cloud allowing instant access at any time.

Competing on the basis of convenience takes tremendous commitment and continuous hard work to stay ahead of competitors. Also, convenience strategies can be expensive. Keeping customer checkout lines short may require pharmacy managers to increase staffing or purchase new technology. Hiring pharmacists to work extended hours can necessitate higher salaries. Pharmacies may find the cost of many convenience strategies to be prohibitive.

Finally, reliance on convenience strategies can have a negative impact on the professional image of pharmacists. High-volume, low-service pharmacies can hurt the public's perception of the professional effort that goes into filling each prescription. Drive-through pharmacies may lead consumers to associate pharmacists more with fast food restaurants than with health care services. Little research is available regarding the impact of convenience strategies on pharmacist image—but think about how consumers would view physicians if they provided consultations at a drive-through window.

Conducting a Convenience Audit

Pharmacy employees and managers need to understand consumer perceptions of the convenience of their business. They need to see the pharmacy as consumers see it. Each pharmacist should be able to answer the following questions about the business:

- How easy it is to enter the parking lot by foot and by car?
- How long does it take to get from the parking lot to the door?
- How long does it take to get from the door to the pharmacy department?
- What obstacles do customers face between the parking lot and the pharmacy department?
- How long is the wait at the pharmacy at different times of the day?
- How many times does the telephone ring before an employee answers it?
- How difficult is it to reach the pharmacist by telephone?
- How long does it take before the automated telephone answering system connects to a human being?
- How often does the pharmacy run out of stock?
- How often do customers ask for items the pharmacy does not stock?
- How many different ways can a patient reach a pharmacist?

In attempting to answer these questions, it is important for pharmacists to act as if they have never been in the pharmacy. For example, trying to maneuver through the store by using only the signage can help identify signs that are unclear and confusing.

SHOPPER MARKETING STRATEGY

Shopper marketing is common strategy in retail pharmacy. *Shopper marketing* is a strategy which seeks to understand how consumers shop and the ways they shop (e.g., online, in-store) to use this information to better compete for their business.[12]

Shopper marketing tries to move from simple transactions at the checkout counter to an *overall experience* where the retailer interacts with the shopper at numerous touchpoints -- smart phone, newspaper circular, store signage, and face-to-face communications. The goal is still to sell merchandise but to do it in way that may be more than utilitarian in nature. Well known masters of this strategy are the Apple Store and Starbucks.

Shopper marketing occurs within the physical store and outside of the store. The experience outside of the store can be physical (e.g., parking lot, billboards) or virtual (e.g., social media, Internet). The overall experience is made up of a series of touchpoints with customers.

For a CVS store visit,[13] initial experiences can occur when customers see the chain's weekly circulars. Circulars can be sent directly to a customer via text, e-mail, or mail and based upon shoppers past purchases and preferences. Once in the store, consumers can use various CVS mobile apps to guide them through the pharmacy. Also, they can use signage or conversations with employees to assist their in-store experience. After leaving the store, they can keep in touch with CVS via various forms of messaging set to their individual preferences regarding type (e.g., discount coupons), channel (e.g., text), and frequency (e.g., weekly).

In pharmacy shopper marketing:

- o The physical pharmacy is a key element of the strategy. The pharmacy is the place where instant purchases are made, and it is a channel preferred by many over internet and mail order.

- o Shopper marketing requires understanding things from the shopper's point-of-view. It needs to offer solutions in multiple channels and communicate with shoppers in numerous ways. Pharmacists can provide insight to the shopper's perspective.

- o Pharmacist services can contribute positively to the shopping experience. They should be coordinated with other shopping initiatives and communication strategies.

MARKETING IN ACTION

Duane Reade's Makeover

Duane Reade is a chain of pharmacies, located in the New York City area which is known for its high volume small store layouts. Now a subsidiary of the Walgreen Company, it was facing big problems prior to 2010. Former company leaders were in jail for financial improprieties, the pharmacies were ranked dead last in customer satisfaction surveys, and stores frequently received low health grades. Complaints about the store were displayed on the "I Hate Duane Reade" blog, and photos of the under stocked, overcrowded store were a viral internet hit. An article in the 2007 New York Magazine wrote, "The dead-eyed pharmacy people at Duane Reade ... It's always a journey into the heart of darkness."

Things have changed since being purchased by Walgreens. A redesign of the store and the merchandizing has changed Duane Reade from an ordeal to a destination. It is said to look as much like a designer store as a pharmacy. Customers can move down well-lit, wide aisles to shop for designer brands. Using the tag line, "Your City. Your Drugstore."; the chain offers a unique New York style experience.

The flagship stores offer an array of services and merchandise. A four-star (out of five stars) Yelp reviewer described a store this way:

"Things this Duane Reade has:

-A juice bar with fresh fruits and vegetables

-A full-service salon where I witnessed a client getting a blowout

-A nail salon with a punch card system (your 6th manicure is free)

-A sparkling and brightly-lit pharmacy with a real waiting area equipped with TVs

-A consultation room within said pharmacy, with sliding doors for privacy

-Tons of staff walking around and helping you find what you're looking for

-Typical pharmacy/DR items such as first aid, shampoo, body wash, lotions, etc.

-A Sephora type makeup room full of department store makeup brands

-Multiple cash registers in different parts of the store

-Tons of FRESH food options to choose from if you want a quick lunch

-A coffee station along with freshly-made doughnuts

**I only chopped off a star because the first sales associate asked what we were looking for, we said Burt's Bees, and she had no idea what that was."

Not all Duane Reade stores have these services but they all seek to provide the same brand service. The brand is boosted by its social media presence. Reviewed in blogs, twitter feeds, and other social media, the chain encourages buzz with contests like the "VIP NYC Bloggers" contest where winners receive $200 a month in store credit in exchange for blogging, tweeting, and Facebooking their love for the store. Coordinating with public relations outreach, Duane Reade invests a large amount of time and effort attracting digital consumers, most of whom are happy to say good things about the store.

Source: Reference [14]

Shopper marketing sees pharmacy purchases as occurring in a retail ecosystem where shoppers travel in search of their needs and desires. Pharmacy communications and services are integrated to address the shoppers' needs anytime, anywhere, and any way. Retailing is less of a visit to a 'pharmacy' and more of a complex sets of actions in which retailers, including pharmacies, come into contact with shoppers.

Shopper marketing is causing pharmacies to rethink the way they do business. Bricks and mortar shopping at pharmacies is changing and pharmacists are adapting. Pharmacists now work with customers to co-create their shopping experiences according to their individual needs. Employees are expected to deliver exceptional service, because service is essential for competing in the market place. And all of this being done in a seamless and convenient manner. Below are some major retail and business trends associated with shopper marketing:[12,13,15]

1) Omnichannel retailing

Omnichannel retailing is an integrated sales experience that combines the advantages of brick-and-mortar stores with benefits of online shopping.[12] Omnichannel retailing tries to integrate the benefits of the store like face-to-face interactions with caring employees with the benefits of online retailing such as infinite choice, rich product information, social media engagement, price comparisons, and the convenience of anything, anytime, anywhere.

2) Branded Service Encounters

Pharmacy employees are a key element in giving customers a reason to visit a physical pharmacy instead of going online. Great employees can give customers branded experiences[16] where they enhance the pharmacy brand by giving exceptional service. A single pharmacist who connects with customers in meaningful ways can drive word-of-mouth recommendations and continued loyalty. Employees like this drive customer visits to stores and even online sales.

3) Using Big Data

Big data, collected from social media, purchase data, and other sources can help pharmacists and pharmacy employees use evidence-based algorithmic recommendations to serve their customers. The possibilities are pretty amazing. Smartphone apps can use geomapping to let retailers know when a customer is approaching a pharmacy's front door and send special offers to them as they enter. Heat-mapping and motion sensors can observe shoppers' movements within a store to learn about their habits and product decisions. In-store Wi-Fi connections can allow mobile phones to communicate with smart shelves that communicate information about specific products on the shelves. Data from millions of visits can be crunched and used to form decision algorithms that employees can use.

4) Decision Support

Retailers are trying to help customers feel supported in their purchase decisions. For example, the Walgreens website offers a digital health advisor to help people reach their health goals, guidance on Medicare Part D, help in finding a local pharmacist using an online search engine, and other services to help support decisions about shopping and health.

5) The Pharmacy as a Community Center

The pharmacy has long been a community center in many towns. This trend is continuing at many stores where pharmacists are asserting their roles as important members of the community. They do things like open their stores to hold yoga classes or participate in health fairs. Connecting with the culture and community of a town generates goodwill and solidifies the health care role of pharmacists.

6) Selling Experiences Not Merchandise

Pharmacy merchandise is becoming increasingly commoditized where price competition is intense. Differentiation in retail comes less from the merchandise sold and more from the experience of customers as they try to fulfill their needs. Building experiences that center around both cognitive and emotional needs of customers can help them understand the value of pharmacists and feel that the pharmacist cares about them too.

7) Low or No Inventory

Retailers like WalMart and Amazon are experimenting with same day and same hour shipping of orders which will reduce the need for store inventory. Zero inventory paves the way for smaller store formats similar to the personalized mom-and-pop stores that used to be the norm in pharmacy practice before the rise of super stores and chains.

8) No Checkout Counter

Waiting in line at the checkout is becoming an outdated ritual with the widespread availability of smartphones. Smart devices can be used by staff to checkout customers anywhere in the store. Sales associates at Walgreens flagship stores can use I-Pads to help customers find what they want and even act as a checkout location if desired. As digital payments become more accepted, customers will be able to make a purchase with the wave of a smartphone, and money will be transferred from the customers' bank account to the pharmacy's. When data from smartphone purchases are paired with a Customer Relationship Management (CRM) system, retailers can customize experiences to customer preferences (e.g., home delivery, notification of discounts). As systems mature, the need for a checkout counter will be rendered obsolete.

ETHICAL MARKETING STRATEGIES

I will hold myself and my colleagues to the
highest principles of our profession's moral,
ethical and legal conduct

-From the Oath of a Pharmacist

Pharmacists face a minefield of potential problems in how they market their services. By necessity, pharmacists must make choices of whom they will serve and how. Some of their choices might be ethically indefensible such as denying access to needy populations who cannot pay, providing poor service to the underserved and unprofitable, and emphasizing profits over care.

Pharmacists can and should be ethical in how they market their products and services because it is good business. Marketing practices that are seen as ethical can improve the image of a firm, enhance consumer trust, increase satisfaction, and make customers more likely to do business with the firm.

Marketers need to use an ethical framework to guide their decisions. One way is to use the following questions to assess the ethics of their strategies.

1. Would I be embarrassed to describe my actions to friends, family members, or professional colleagues?
2. How would I feel if a marketer acted in a similar manner toward me?
3. How would an objective jury of my peers judge my actions?
4. Does the strategy benefit my customers less than, as much as, or more than it benefits me?
5. Is the strategy consistent with our firm's mission and ethics code?

6. Am I taking advantage of a population that is vulnerable because of age, education, income, language, or some other factor?
7. Do consumers have sufficient knowledge to make a good decision?
8. Are consumers free to choose another provider if I do not serve them well?

SUMMARY

Pharmacists have traditionally relied on a limited number of strategies for marketing their services. This chapter presents several new strategies to consider.

Reference List

(1) Kauffman V, Tsouderos T. The Future of Health is More, Better, Cheaper. Strategy and Business [78]. 2-2-2015.

(2) Buss D. Walgreens Promotes Digital Health With Wearable Tech, Virtual Doctor Visits. Brand Channel . 12-8-2014. 2-16-2015.

(3) Garrison LP, Jr., Veenstra DL. The economic value of innovative treatments over the product life cycle: the case of targeted trastuzumab therapy for breast cancer. Value Health 2009;12(8):1118-1123.

(4) Krentz SE, Pilskaln SM. Product life cycle: still a valid framework for business planning. Top Health Care Financ 1988;15(1):40-48.

(5) Schommer JC, Doucette WR, Johnson KA, Planas LG. Positioning and integrating medication therapy management. J Am Pharm Assoc (2003) 2012;52(1):12-24.

(6) Brown D, Portlock J, Rutter P, Nazar Z. From community pharmacy to healthy living pharmacy: positive early experiences from Portsmouth, England. Res Social Adm Pharm 2014;10(1):72-87.

(7) Patterson BJ, Doucette WR, Urmie JM, McDonough RP. Exploring relationships among pharmacy service use, patronage motives, and patient satisfaction. J Am Pharm Assoc (2003) 2013;53(4):382-389.

(8) Franic DM, Haddock SM, Tucker LT, Wooten N. Pharmacy patronage: identifying key factors in the decision making process using the determinant attribute approach. J Am Pharm Assoc (2003) 2008;48(1):71-85.

(9) Dominelli A, Weck MM, Jarvis J. Service preferences differences between community pharmacy and supermarket pharmacy patrons. Health Mark Q 2005;23(1):57-79.

(10) Goad JA, Taitel MS, Fensterheim LE, Cannon AE. Vaccinations administered during off-clinic hours at a national community pharmacy: implications for increasing patient access and convenience. Ann Fam Med 2013;11(5):429-436.

(11) Liberman JN, Girdish C. Recent trends in the dispensing of 90-day-supply prescriptions at retail pharmacies: implications for improved convenience and access. Am Health Drug Benefits 2011;4(2):95-100.

(12) Rigby D. The future of shopping. Harvard Business Review 2011;89(12):65-76.

(13) PSFK. The Future of Retail 2015: A Manafesto to Reinvent the Retail Store. New York, NY: PSFK; 2015.

(14) Grant D. The Re-Education of Duane Reade: A Drugstore as Retail, Therapy. New York Observer 2013 Apr 23.

(15) Sorescu A, Frambach RT, Singh J, Rangaswamy A, Bridges C. Innovations in Retail Business Models. Journal of Retailing 2011;87, Supplement 1(0):S3-S16.

(16) Sirianni NJ, Bitner MJ, Brown SW, Mandel N. Branded service encounters: Strategically aligning employee behavior with the brand positioning. Journal of Marketing 2013;77(6):108-123.

Chapter Questions

1. Can pharmacists use both cost and differentiation strategies in marketing their services? Explain your answer.

2. Name one pharmacy service or merchandise item that you think is in each phase of the product life cycle: introduction, growth, maturity, and decline.

3. What is gained and lost when pharmacists adopt convenience strategies?

4. Identify a business that you think does a good job with shopper marketing. What strategies do they use to offer a great shopping experience? Can these strategies be used in pharmacies?

Activities

1. Go to an independent or chain pharmacy Web site. Write a short paragraph summarizing how the pharmacy positions itself in the market using various elements of the marketing mix (i.e., the four P's). What products and services make up its strategic portfolio? How would you describe its overall portfolio strategy?

2. Conduct a convenience audit of a pharmacy or other business that you frequent. What recommendations would you make to improve the convenience of the business?

CHAPTER **6**

INNOVATION STRATEGIES

Objectives

After studying this chapter, the reader should be able to

- o   Define what is an innovation
- o   Describe how pharmacies and pharmacists innovate
- o   Contrast red and blue ocean strategies
- o   Suggest ways that pharmacists can serve customers in innovative ways

If you always do what you always did, you will always get what you always got.

- Albert Einstein

An *innovation* is any change in the marketing mix that customers perceive as new. It can be a change in products, services, or processes. Customers adopt innovations for a complex mix of reasons, including the relative benefits it provide over competing products, the ease with which an innovation can be incorporated into the customer's life, and the perceived risk of adopting it.[1] Innovations can be used to

- Find new customers for a product (e.g., expand pharmacy services to customers with pets)

- Find new uses for a product (e.g., use superglue to close wounds)

- Increase usage of existing products (e.g., offer a customer loyalty card)

- Expand a product line (e.g., offer disease management in addition to basic dispensing services)

- Expand distribution intensity (e.g., increase the number of pharmacies in an area)

- Expand distribution over a wider geographic area (e.g., expand into new geographic markets)

- Penetrate the markets of competitors (e.g., develop a service that will draw away a competitor's target customers)

INNOVATION IN PHARMACY

Pharmacy practice is not typically very innovative. Most changes in practice are incremental, such as a new computer program, the reorganization of a pharmacy layout, a coupon promotion plan, or a change in the work process. Many such changes are not really innovations, but imitations of competitor strategies. This makes many pharmacies appear very similar to customers. Indeed, most pharmacies are alike--having similar merchandise, services, layout, and overall atmosphere. Most use a similar business strategies consisting of some variation of low pricing and one-stop shopping convenience.

Lack of innovation in marketing strategies is common in many industries. Kim and Mauborgne[1] state that this is because competitors "share a conventional wisdom about who their customers are and what they value, and about the scope of products and services their industry should be offering." When a majority of businesses within an industry share the same conventional wisdom, they end up competing in essentially the same way.

MARKETING IN ACTION

Seeing a solution that pharmacists could not

Sometimes it takes outsiders to see solutions that people in a profession cannot. For instance, Deborah Adler was getting a masters degree in Design at the School of Visual Arts, in New York City. Her grandmother mistakenly took her grandfather's medication for her own because of the similarities in their respective prescription bottles. Although the results could have been tragic, her grandmother was not hurt.

Still, this error had a profound effect on her and led to developing a new prescription bottle for her thesis project. Pharmacists had been using the same amber-colored bottle design since the mid 20th century despite problems with legibility of directions, similarities in bottles, and other challenges for consumers. She designed a solution to address these challenges.

Her thesis resulted in the ClearRx system, a nationally available prescription system at Target. Using color coded rings to identify each family member and easy-to-read labels, the ClearRx innovation did not come from pharmacists, who were so used to the old bottle designs that they never really questioned their use. The ClearRx innovation required someone outside of the pharmacy profession to make it happen.

Source: Reference [2]

One reason that many pharmacies and pharmacists are similar is that the professional educational system does not often encourage creativity and innovation in students. Although professional education is evolving, students are still trained to be compliant in how they behave inside and outside of class, get THE correct answer on exams, and not take chances in graded assignments that might jeopardize high grades. Students recruited for pharmacy schools predominantly come from basic science background which tends to reinforce a rigidity of thinking and approach to pharmacy practice.

Another reason for the lack of innovation in pharmacy practice is that innovating can be risky and hard work. In the short term, it is usually safer and easier to copy the practices of competitors than to take risks on new ideas. People rarely get fired for following the crowd, but they often are terminated for taking chances. Innovating also requires companies and people to change and establish new ways of doing business. Resistance to change can be a reasonable response to taking chances, especially when the old way is still profitable. And finally, many new products and services fail in the market along with the careers of people who have promoted them.

A casual review of pharmacy trade magazines shows that most pharmacies follow a similar set of strategies: convenience, low price, emphasis on the pharmacist, merchandise variety, and niche marketing. Innovations in pharmacy generally result from improvements in operational efficiency, operational effectiveness, governance, and convenience/access (Table 6-1).[3]

Table 6-1: Pharmacy Innovations

Innovation Classification	Examples
Greater Operational Efficiency	Delegating Tasks To Techs and Robotic technologies
	Self-checkout Technology
	Mail Order/Internet Pharmacy/Drive-thru
	Touch Screen Interactive Kiosks
	Electronic Refill Reminders/Electronic Prescribing
	ATM-like Dispensing Machines
	Specialization Of Tasks (e.g., MTM, specialty medicines)
Enhanced Operational Effectiveness	Targeting Specific Customer Segments (e.g., seniors, diabetes)
	Medication Synchronization
	MTM/ Disease Management/Case Management
	Office-based Pharmacy
	Pharmacists Embedded in Health Care Teams and Medical Homes
	Public Health Services/Immunizations
	Specialty Pharmacy
	OTC/Complementary Medicine Counseling
	Smartphone Apps
	Customer Relationship Management (CRM) Systems
	Coordinated Pharmacy & Retail Clinic Services
Locking in Customers	Pharmacy Benefit Management Contracts
	Rx Benefit Adjudication & Services
	Limited Pharmacy Networks
	Mandatory/Preferred Mail Order Pharmacy Contracts
	Customer Loyalty Cards
	Store Membership (e.g., Costco, Sam's Warehouse)
	Medication Synchronization
	MTM/Disease Management
	Customer Relationship Management (CRM) Systems
	Exclusive Retailers of Desirable Brands (e.g., Store brands)
Improved Governance	Independent Pharmacy Groups (E.G., Good Neighbor)
	Independent Pharmacy Franchises (E.G., Health Mart, Medicine Shoppe)
	Group Purchasing Organizations
	Professional Associations
	Internet Only Pharmacies
	Pharmacies Within Integrated Health Systems
	Physician Owned/Contracted Pharmacies
	Pharmacy Benefit Managers
More Convenience/ Access	Numerous Variations On One-Stop-Shopping
	Drive Thru/Online/Mail Order/Self-Service
	Online Access To Locations & Individual Store Maps
	Omni-Channel Retailing
	Clearly Marked Merchandise And Prices
	Good Store Layout & Easy Traffic Flow In The Aisles
	Minimal Out-Of-Stock Merchandise
	Expanded Operating Hours
	Clinic Pharmacies In Or Next To Physicians' Offices & Hospitals

Greater Operational Efficiency. These innovations describe how pharmacy practice is made faster, cheaper, and/or simpler. It involves providing value more with minimal additional resources and waste. The pharmacy literature is filled with recommendations and case studies about how pharmacists can be more efficient by streamlining front end and back end workflow, managing personnel and inventory, utilizing new technology, and reducing costs of providing care.

Enhanced Operational Effectiveness. Improving operational effectiveness means meeting the needs of customers better. It differs from operational efficiency which refers to serving customers faster, cheaper, and/or simpler. Effectiveness means serving customers according to their individualized needs. In pharmacy practice, it might mean spending extra time and effort on patients with complex medication related problems rather than dispensing medications quickly and efficiently without regard to how they are taken or the health outcomes received. Examples of operational effectiveness in pharmacy include the provision of MTM services, offering immunization services, and appointment based medication synchronization.

Locking In Customers. This innovation is intended to reduce customer churn (i.e., frequent switching of pharmacy providers). Linked to relationship marketing strategies, the goal is to increase the costs of switching either by charging more for leaving the relationship or giving more so customers will not want to switch. Examples in pharmacy include contracts with pharmacy benefit managers, customer relationship management programs, and appointment based medication synchronization.

Lock-in strategies are controversial because they can be seen as anticompetitive (e.g., restricted pharmacy networks). This has led to legislation regulating their use (e.g., any willing provider laws). Nevertheless, they are increasingly used as a cost control measure in managing pharmaceutical expenses.

Improved Governance. Governance describes the processes and structures that organizations use to coordinate and control how they serve customers. Governance occurs at various levels within (e.g., department, store, corporation) and between organizations (e.g., Accountable Care Organization, HMO). Examples of governance innovations include structures that encourage cooperation among entities like independent pharmacy groups and franchises, professional associations which advocate for pharmacists and serve other member needs, and health system structures like pharmacies that contract with health systems to provide integrated care.

More Convenience/Access. Convenience innovations improve the ability of customers to access to medications and are key strategies for pharmacies. Most pharmacy innovations, like online and drive-thru pharmacies, attempt to make drugs available any time or place. Examples include Omni-channel retailing and technological innovations like online, self-service, and mobile solutions.

The innovations in Table 6-1 have significant benefits for pharmacy customers, but many are easy for competitors to imitate. Consequently, they offer little sustainable competitive advantage. The advantage gained by the first drive thru pharmacy was quickly dissipated because the innovation was easy to copy by competitors and quickly became standard in US pharmacies. In many cases, sustainable competitive advantage occurs through the people and processes that accompany the service innovations because excellent service design and performance is hard to duplicate. Exceptional, highly engaged employees in well designed pharmacies can offer personalized, unique service experiences.

BLUE OCEAN INNOVATIONS

The idea behind Blue Ocean innovations is that success in the marketplace can occur by creating demand in uncontested, unrecognized markets.[4] Rather that compete head-to-head with people offering the same mix of services and merchandise ("Red Ocean"), pharmacists can compete in markets that are uncontested and unrecognized ("Blue Ocean").

Red Oceans in community pharmacy practice today consist of the dispensing of drugs in retail settings. In these red ocean pharmacies, pharmacists have clearly defined boundaries of their roles, and they do not step outside of those restrictions. Pharmacists compete for the same pool of customers using similar services and merchandise. The primary way of winning is to provide these services and merchandise faster and cheaper than rival pharmacists and thereby grab a greater share of available patients. In red oceans, however, competition increases over time and everyone begins to resemble each other -- matching strategies in order to compete. In these markets, products and services become commodities and fierce competition turns the ocean (i.e., market) bloody or red.

On the other hand, blue oceans describe open, unknown, and poorly served market spaces. The term, "blue ocean" is used as an analogy of the unexplored market space. In blue oceans, opportunities are explored -- unencumbered by competition. An example in health care is the retail medical clinic, which at one time had sole ownership of a major part of the ambulatory healthcare market. Now, the market is becoming redder and redder.

With an open mind and good imagination, pharmacists can identify new blue ocean opportunities with the following advice.

1. Differentiate yourself from direct competitors
2. Get ideas for indirect competitors
3. Provide simpler alternatives
4. Look at participants other than the end user
5. Provide complimentary products and services
6. Go beyond functional appeal

1. DIFFERENTIATE YOURSELF FROM DIRECT COMPETITORS

Innovative pharmacists continually look for ways to differentiate themselves from direct competitors who offer similar products and services (see intratype competitors in Chapter 2). Rather than mimicking the innovations of these direct competitors, pharmacists could do things differently. For instance, they can quit thinking about the tangible product (i.e., drug) and focus on the health care experience. Instead of the typical pharmacy visit where the patient gets in and out as quickly as possible, a pharmacy could concentrate on being a desirable destination where people can explore health-related products and services. A pharmacy in Boulder, Colorado, has done this.[5]

Pharmaca Integrative Pharmacy integrates natural remedies, herbal supplements, and alternative therapies with modern medical practices and prescription drug therapies. Shoppers are treated to light jazz or classical background music, scents from aromatherapy candles, and subdued lighting from strategically placed track lights. Contrast that with the typical community pharmacy that uses bright fluorescent lighting, Muzak, and a traditional merchandise mix.

"Design Thinking" is one strategy used to differentiate businesses.[6] Design Thinking is a method popularized by the design company IDEO that describes a process of immersing oneself into the context of a problem (e.g., medication non-adherence), creatively generating insights and solutions (e.g., new devices, apps, or services), and designing technologically feasible and workable business models for success.

The premise of Design Thinking is that processes commonly utilized by design companies can effectively solve difficult, complex problems using the following general steps:[7]

- o **Define**: Identify the target audience and choose measures to evaluate success.
- o **Research**: Immerse yourself into the history of existing obstacles. Speak with end-users to gather insight and ideas about needs of end-users for further development.
- o **Ideate**: Create many potential solutions to serve the needs of end-users for future testing.
- o **Prototype**: Expand and refine ideas, create multiple drafts, and seek feedback from a diverse group of end-users.
- o **Choose**: Review the objective, set aside emotion and ownership of ideas, avoid consensus thinking, and select the powerful ideas.
- o **Implement**: Make task descriptions, determine resources, and execute the plan.
- o **Learn**: Test ideas in markets, learn from mistakes, make changes, and test again.

Design Thinking has been used to develop pharmacist services.[7-9] Walgreens used it to design flagship stores in locations across the US which feature the new "Wellness Experience" format. In the Wellness Experience format pharmacists have an expanded role in managing patient care. Pharmacists are located at an "Ask Your Pharmacist" desk instead of behind the counter filling prescriptions. Pharmacists triage patients to either the pharmacy or primary care clinic. Counseling and MTM is conducted in private consultation rooms and pharmacists are encouraged to engage in providing the care they have been trained to do.

Design Thinking has been used to help implement MTM services in community pharmacies.[7] The process was used to gain insight into consumer thinking and offer new ways of providing and communicating about MTM. For example, they discovered the critical importance of physicians in the promotion and success of MTM. "The most success we had in our personal marketing approach was going right to the physicians and getting them to promote our services. Simply by convincing them that MTM is an important part of care."[7] Design Thinking can be used to identify solutions to numerous patient needs in the community (Figure 6-1).

Figure 6-1 Patient Needs That Can Be Addressed with Design Thinking by Community Pharmacists

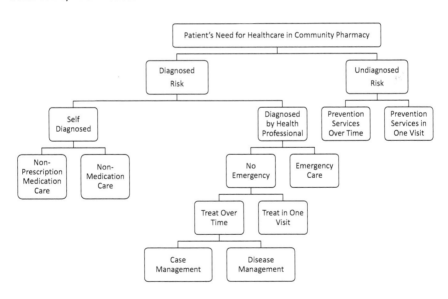

2. GET IDEAS FROM INDIRECT COMPETITORS

Pharmacists looking for innovations can also get ideas from intertype competitors; those who provide distinctly different products that indirectly compete by meeting similar customer needs and wants (see Chapter 2). Consumers choose products and services that they think will solve their problems. They are less interested in what is provided than in how well it meets their needs.

Consumers may consider products and services from many different industries to meet their needs. A person who is interested in an evening of entertainment might choose from the film, television, theater, restaurant, or sporting industries. Similarly, a person who catches a cold might choose from chicken soup (food industry), cold medicine (pharmaceutical industry), Echinacea (herbal industry), or a visit to a physician (medical services industry).

Pharmacists who want to identify new solutions to patient problems need to study how consumers make these choices. Table 6-2 shows the steps involved in choices for treating a cold. Each choice results in different actions and outcomes. When patients go to a physician for a cold, they must make an appointment, go to the office, wait for the physician to become available, get a prescription or other treatment recommendation, go to a pharmacy, wait while the prescription is filled, and finally go home to take the medication. After going through this process, the patient may receive some symptomatic relief, but the cold will not resolve faster than with any of the other options.

Table 6.2 Consumer Choices for Treating a Cold

Options	Steps	Outcome
Go to a physician	1. Make an appointment and go to the office. 2. Get a prescription. 3. Have the prescription filled at a pharmacy.	Significant time and effort spent. The condition resolves itself in approximately the same time as it would with other options. Some symptomatic relief possible. The patient is assured that the cold is not something else.
Choose a cold medicine	1. Go to a pharmacy or other store that stocks nonprescription medications. 2. Decide among various nonprescription choices.	Some time and effort required to go to the store. If the customer is unfamiliar with the choices, he or she must seek assistance from store personnel. The customer may be concerned about adverse effects or drug interactions. Some symptomatic relief possible.

Choose an herbal product	1. Go to a pharmacy or other store that stocks herbal medicines. 2. Decide among various herbal choices.	Some time and effort required to go to the store. If the customer is unfamiliar with the choices, he or she must seek assistance from store personnel. The customer may inappropriately feel safe from adverse effects and drug interactions.
Treat with food	1. Go to the kitchen cupboard. 2. Open a can of chicken soup.	Minimal time, effort, and money spent. May be reminded about how colds were treated during childhood and feel some comfort.

Many people are too busy to visit a physician for a cold, so they choose self-treatment that may be as efficacious as a physician visit, without the time and expense. They might choose nonprescription medications, herbal products, or food.

Self-treatment carries its own risks. The patient may be suffering from a more serious condition that needs medical treatment. What might appear to be a cold could actually be pneumonia or some other serious infection. Self-treatment also carries the risk of adverse effects and interactions with prescribed drugs.

The patient's options have different perceived costs and benefits. Some of those perceptions are based on false assumptions e.g., non-prescription and herbal drugs are completely safe. Pharmacists are in an excellent position to help the patient with the selection process. In fact, many already do. However, pharmacists can do much more.[10] They can encourage patients to discuss their options. Patient–pharmacist communication can be enhanced if the pharmacist is readily available and on the lookout for consumers who are in need.

Communication can also be enhanced through good shelf displays. During cold season, the pharmacist can display a brochure or sign that delineates the most common options for treating a cold and the consequences associated with each option. The display could grab customer attention with pictures of a physician, a nonprescription medication, an herbal product, and a can of chicken soup above discussions of each option. Good displays can educate consumers about treatment alternatives and direct them to the pharmacist if necessary.

3. PROVIDE SIMPLER ALTERNATIVES

In its efforts to continually offer more expensive, technologically demanding innovations, the US health care system tends to overshoot the needs of the vast majority of patients. Most illnesses that afflict patients are generally uncomplicated and easily resolved with basic diagnoses and treatments. However, health care education, physician specialists, pharmaceutical companies, and hospitals continually seek to meet the needs of the most demanding, complex, and difficult to cure patients. Much less effort is being spent on meeting the needs of the vast majority of patients who seek solutions that are simpler, more convenient, and less costly.

The overemphasis by dominant players in health care on complex, high-cost innovations provides an opportunity for disruptive innovations to fill the gap.[11, 12] Disruptive innovations succeed by enabling people to substitute simpler solutions for more complex, expensive options. Examples in health care include the substitution of nurse practitioners for general practitioners and specialists, patient self-care for physician-directed care, and vaccinations at pharmacies instead of physicians' offices. Disruptive innovations compete by filling the gap left by businesses that focus on serving the profitable upscale market. Opportunities are found to serve the low-end market with products of slightly lower quality (but good enough) that are simpler, cheaper, and/or more convenient.

Disruptive innovations occur in medicine.[11, 12] Health care services exist in a hierarchy of increasing complexity ranging from self-care providers (pharmacists, herbalists) to physician specialists (allergists, dermatologists). As specialists focus on treating the sickest patients, less-skilled but competent providers can take on more complex roles that they had never attempted before. Family practitioners take on diagnostic and treatment tasks that were once only within the domain of specialists. Nurse practitioners and physician assistants diagnose and treat conditions that used to be performed solely by family practitioners. Drugs that used to be prescription only can now be purchased over-the-counter along with self-diagnostic devices for diabetes, cholesterol, blood pressure, and pregnancy. The move toward consumer directed health care and improvements in technology will continue to drive this trend.

Pharmacists have been participants and recipients of disruptive innovation (Table 6.3). They have disrupted physician practice by selling self-treatments and self-diagnostic products -- meeting the needs of patients who might have visited doctors' offices. Pharmacists have also disrupted by providing vaccinations, specialty medicine services, and various disease management services that were once the sole territory of physicians.

Table 6-3 Examples of Disruptive Innovations in Pharmacy Practice

Disruptor	Disruptee
Pharmacists - disrupting physician practice by selling self-diagnostics and self-treatments, vaccinations, specialty medicine services, and disease management.	Physicians
Technology and pharmacy technicians - disrupt traditional dispensing roles	Dispensing pharmacists
Pharmacy Chains - disrupt the community model with low prices and nationwide access to prescriptions	Local Independents
Distant pharmacist service through online and mail order - disrupt - disrupt the requirement that face-to-face services are needed for all prescriptions	Face-to-face pharmacist service at brick-and-mortar pharmacies
Do-it-yourself pharmacy technology with apps and ATM-like medication dispensing - disrupt the need for pharmacists to be in control	Pharmacist participation in the medication use process

Pharmacists have also been on the receiving end of disruptive innovations. Pharmacist roles have been disrupted by technology and pharmacy technicians. Retail pharmacy models have been disrupted by competitors who offer lower prices and greater convenience. Potential future disruptors might be ATM-dispensing machines in physicians' offices which are seen as an alternative to pharmacy visits. Some patients may decide to sacrifice the value of pharmacist services for the convenience of one-stop treatment of their medical needs.

MARKETING IN ACTION

Grow your own drugs

James Wong is an ethnobotanist, trained at the Royal Botanic Gardens in London, who promotes the idea of growing your own drugs. He has written a medicinal recipe book titled Grow Your Own Drugs and he has a BBC television series with that name.

Wong's interest is in getting people to grow their own pharmacy of herbal medicines in their backyards: drugs like fennel, rose hips, Echinacea, aloe vera, chilies, blue berries, and dandelion.

He thinks that people suffer from "Plant Prejudice", where they have stereotyped ideas about herbal medicines. He sees plants as little chemical factories and argues that people draw a big black line between conventional, scientific medicine and natural plant-based medicine. To him, this bias is based upon cultural bias, not science. To Wong, the main difference is the packaging-- modern medicine is packaged in pills and natural medicine comes in the cells of plants.

Wong's book, BBC series, and website promote remedies for a wide range of ailments — from eczema to sore throats to hot flashes to head lice. He recommends that these remedies should be used for minor ailments or only after traditional medicine fails.

Wong counsels people to be responsible experimenters. This means knowing the drugs you are using and do not self-diagnosing. Even the best therapies do not work if they are used for the wrong diagnoses.

His website offers herbal solutions for a range of conditions including:

- o Head lice - Neem oil, produced from a subtropical tree, native to India which is widely available and inexpensively in health food shops

- o Athlete's foot - a garlic footbath of garlic, sage leaves, cider, and vinegar

- o Irritable bowel syndrome, indigestion, or heartburn -- peppermint tea

Wong points out that all of the herbs and plants he recommends have a long history of use and no record of toxicity. If traditional medicine isn't working, why not try herbals.

Sources: National Public Radio, www.jameswong.co.uk

4. LOOK AT PARTICIPANTS OTHER THAN THE END USER

Ideas for innovations can come from thinking about participants other than the end user (i.e., the patient). Patients rarely make purchasing decisions about health care products and services without help from others (Table 6-4).

The patient may be the one who takes medication or receives treatment, but the decider is often a physician, not the patient. The physician chooses a treatment for the patient, and the patient is expected to follow the physician's directions.

Third-party payers, such as insurance companies, employers, and the government, also influence treatment choice. Third-party payers may exert influence through copayment policies, prior-authorization programs, and formularies. Other times, they act as deciders by refusing to pay for specific treatments.

Additional parties who influence health care decision-making include nurses, pharmacists, employers, family members, and friends. Depending on the situation, they can take on a variety of roles in the purchase process. Pharmacists who understand the roles played by each party in diverse situations can identify new market opportunities.

TABLE 6-4 Participants in the Health Care Purchase Process

Decision-Making Role	Examples
End User	Patients
Decider	Physicians, patient, family members, payers, pharmacists, nurses, managed care plans, government (laws, rules), pharmacy benefit managers, employers and others who pay for health insurance
Influencer	Physicians, patient, family members, payers, pharmacists, nurses, pharmaceutical industry, managed care plans, wholesalers, government (laws, rules), pharmacy benefit managers, employers and others who pay for health insurance

The pharmaceutical industry has been very successful over the years in targeting different participants in the drug-use process. They no longer market prescription drugs solely to physician prescribers. They now promote pharmaceuticals to the public, advocacy groups, politicians, health care payers, and anyone else with a role in the purchase process for drugs.

Pharmacists too have learned to target other participants in the drug- use process. They used to market their services almost exclusively to patients, because most patients paid for their medications out of pocket. The spread of prescription drug insurance and the resulting influence of managed care have forced pharmacists to cater to the desires of employer groups, pharmacy benefit managers, managed care companies, and physician groups. In some cases, the consequences have been negative: lowered dispensing fees. In other cases, positive outcomes have occurred, such as contracts with managed care providers to provide disease management services and collaborative practice agreements with physicians to help them manage patient health conditions and control drug costs.

Each party involved in health care decisions has a different definition of value. Finding ways to serve these different customers can offer opportunities for pharmacists.

5. PROVIDE COMPLEMENTARY PRODUCTS AND SERVICES

Pharmaceuticals are often accompanied by complementary or value-added products or services that facilitate the appropriate use of medications. Dispensing services are a complement to physician prescribing services, because they reduce the delivery of inaccurate and dangerous prescription drugs. MTM services complement basic dispensing services, because they reduce drug-related problems.

Pharmacists can identify new opportunities to provide complementary services by first defining the total solution that customers seek when choosing a product or service. Although health is an important outcome of a pharmacy visit, it is not the only one. Many older, retired patients see a visit to the pharmacy as a social outing that gets them out of the house or gives them an opportunity to chat about everyday matters. Some pharmacies encourage the use of the store as a social center by offering café sections or waiting areas where individuals can meet to catch up on local news and converse about topics of interest.

Pharmacists can identify new complementary service opportunities by considering what happens before, during, and after a visit to the pharmacy or other health care provider. They can identify opportunities that add value to the prescription drug process by mapping out all of the steps involved from the time of problem recognition to the time the medical condition is resolved. Consider the following questions:

- When and how do consumers realize they need physician services?
- When and how do consumers realize they need pharmacy services?
- Whom do they consult about their medical conditions?
- What media do they use for health information?
- When, where, and how do consumers decide to seek pharmacy services?
- What issues are important in selecting pharmacy services?
- What problems do consumers have in finding, purchasing, and paying for pharmacy services?
- What problems do consumers have once they have purchased pharmacy products or services?

Answering these questions can offer ideas for easing barriers faced by patients in the drug-use process. Pharmacies can enhance patient problem recognition by creating displays that stimulate curiosity about health topics. Pharmacists can do the same by engaging customers in conversations about health needs and interests. Pharmacies can have a section for health care books. Comfortable seating and even a coffee or snack bar can be provided to make the pharmacy an inviting, pleasant place to go. Pharmacists can improve post-purchase evaluation by inviting patients to discuss problems they have after leaving the pharmacy.

6. GO BEYOND FUNCTIONAL APPEAL

Pharmacists usually promote the functional appeal -- practical issues such as price, location, and quality -- of pharmacy goods and services over their emotional appeal. Pharmacists typically assume that people are thoughtful and rational in their actions. Consequently, they highlight cognitive arguments about the utility of pharmacy products and their value. However, pharmacists may be missing an opportunity.

Other industries recognize the value of emotional appeals to consumers. Cosmetic companies successfully evoke a wide range of emotional images of their products, even though most cosmetics are made up of the same basic ingredients. It is often said that the cosmetics industry sells beauty and hope. If appeals were rational, much of the magic of cosmetics would be lost.

A company's emphasis on functional or emotional appeal sets customers' expectations of the business. Most pharmacies have trained their customers to expect speed, price, and location in the purchase of pharmaceuticals. Pharmacies could challenge the status quo by adding more emotion to the pharmacy shopping experience.

A great deal can be learned from the coffee industry. It has done a wonderful job of taking a functional product and injecting emotion into the consumption process. Functionally, coffee can be promoted on the basis of how hot it is, its freshness, and its cost. But Starbucks and other companies have made coffee drinking into a special event. Whoever would have thought that people would wait in line for the privilege of paying $5 for a steaming solution of coffee beans? Starbucks has changed the coffee shop from a place to buy a cup of coffee to a "caffeine-induced oasis."[1]

Some pharmacies tap into emotion. Those with soda fountains appeal to childhood memories. Other pharmacies emphasize the emotional bonds that exist between pharmacists, patients, and communities. Many small pharmacies appeal to emotions through the unique mix of merchandise they carry. Traditional merchandising rules might not recommend stocking craft supplies, gift items, and even deli supplies in pharmacies. Sometimes a nontraditional mix of merchandise can help small pharmacies compete against large chains. Rather than being just a place to make purchases, they offer a unique shopping experience.

SUMMARY

Pharmacists have traditionally relied on a limited number of strategies for marketing their services. This chapter presents several new strategies to consider.

MARKETING IN ACTION

Developing a New Device to Halt Allergy Attacks

Eric and Evan Edwards are twin brothers from Richmond, Virginia who always need to carry an epinephrine injection device with them wherever they go. They have been doing it since childhood because they have grown up with serious food allergies and were under doctor's orders to carry their medicine everywhere they went. An epinephrine injection device was needed to save them from the life threatening anaphylaxis associated with their food allergies.

As children, they hated carrying around the EpiPen epinephrine device, finding it bulky and difficult to use. Shaped like a large felt tipped marker, they would often forget it at home. On one vacation during their teenage years, they thought they had forgotten to pack their EpiPens. They worried that the trip was ruined until their mother found some extras stored in luggage. That was when they mapped out plans for a new device on a napkin.

The napkin (which they have to this day) contained the first prototype drawings for the Auvi-Q epinephrine injection device with automated voice instructions. The device is slimmer, shaped more like a smartphone than a felt tipped pen, and it talks users though the process of responding to severe allergic reaction. The entry of the Auvi-Q device onto the market in 2013 was the culmination of a 15-year quest of juggling education, family, and business.

In a single-minded journey, the teenaged twins plotted out a strategy to get the education they needed to develop and market their device. Evan went to engineering school at the University of Virginia and Eric became a medical student at Virginia Commonwealth University (VCU). While in med school, Eric took a leave of absence to get his PhD in pharmaceutical sciences at the School of Pharmacy--taking an extensive number of courses ranging from pharmaceutics to pharmaceutical marketing. After completing his PhD, he went back to complete his MD training. All of this was done while being married, raising a family, and volunteering within the community.

Sometime during their education, they started a company called Intelliject (now named Kaleo) to develop their idea. Pitching their idea to friends, family members, venture capitalists, and former pharmaceutical executives, they developed a small team that overcame the numerous hurdles associated with bringing a medical device to market. Their persistence paid off.

The company licensed the product to Sanofi in 2009 for more than $200 million. The Auvi-Q has been in demand among allergy sufferers, who have praised its compact design and "cool" factor. Not being individuals who rest on their accomplishments, the brothers and Kaleo have recently introduced a take-home naloxone auto-injector onto the market for use by patients, family members, and other caregivers in case an opioid overdose occurs.

Sources: New York Times, Eric Edwards

Reference List

(1) Kim WC, Mauborgne R. Creating new market space. Harvard Business Review 1999;77(1):83-+.

(2) Adler D. Adler Design 2014 December 24;Available at: URL: www.adlerdesign.com.

(3) Sorescu A, Frambach RT, Singh J, Rangaswamy A, Bridges C. Innovations in Retail Business Models. Journal of Retailing 2011;87, Supplement 1(0):S3-S16.

(4) Kim WC, Mauborgne R. Blue ocean strategy. Harv Bus Rev 2004;82(10):76-84, 156.

(5) Gentry CR. Health, harmony and higher sales. An ordinary drug store becomes an extraordinary health-and-wellness center. Chain Store Age 77[4], 41. 2001.

(6) Brown T. Design thinking. Harv Bus Rev 2008;86(6):84-92, 141.

(7) Isetts BJ, Schommer JC, Westberg SM, Johnson JK, Froiland NHJM. Evaluation of a Consumer-Generated Marketing Plan for Medication Therapy Management Services . Innovations in Pharmacy 2012;2(1):1-19.

(8) Parker TJ. Prescribing Design. Design Management Review 2014;25(3):30-33.

(9) IDEO. Community Pharmacy for Walgreens. Transforming the corner drugstore into a destination for health and daily living. 2015. 2-12-2015.

(10) Wertheimer AI, Serradell J. A discussion paper on self-care and its implications for pharmacists. Pharm World Sci 2008;30(4):309-315.

(11) Christensen CM, Bohmer R, Kenagy J. Will disruptive innovations cure health care? Harv Bus Rev 2000;78(5):102-12, 199.

(12) Hwang J, Christensen CM. Disruptive innovation in health care delivery: a framework for business-model innovation. Health Aff (Millwood) 2008;27(5):1329-1335.

Chapter Questions

1. What problems might occur when pharmacists copy each other's marketing strategies?

2. What is an innovation? What are the benefits and costs of being highly innovative? What are the risks?

3. What is the biggest problem facing patients in taking their medications? Come up with 10 ideas to solve that problem. When generating your ideas, try to suggest things that have never been tried before or are just crazy. The crazy ideas are often the beginning step to real innovations.

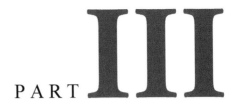

PART **III**

Marketing
Pharmacist Services

CHAPTER 7

CHARACTERISTICS OF SERVICES

Objectives

After studying this chapter, the reader should be able to

- o Define the following terms: services, value-added services, pure services, core services, facilitating services, and supporting services
- o Describe characteristics of services that differentiate them from products
- o Discuss how the characteristics of services make them difficult to market
- o Describe service categorization methods that can be used to develop strategic insights into the provision of pharmacist services
- o List marketing strategies for dealing with the unique characteristics of services

All businesses provide services to some degree. For some businesses, like consulting and insurance, service is the core benefit they provide. For others, like manufacturing and retailing, services are secondary to the sale of merchandise.

In recent years, the practice of pharmacy has been trying to move from being a product-centered profession to one that is a service-centered. This has lead to efforts to redefine the image of pharmacists and pharmacy services in the eyes of patients, the general public, payers, pharmacists, and other health care providers. These efforts have promoted the image that pharmacists provide professional services, not just drugs. A major part of the message is that pharmacist services add value to drug therapy. Without services provided by pharmacists, many drugs can be ineffective and even harmful.

Indeed, pharmacy is fundamentally a service profession. Although often associated with a tangible product, pharmacy practice revolves around the provision of services. In fact, few instances exist in pharmacy practice where services do not accompany a product. Pharmacy services are provided with every prescription, nonprescription, and nondrug product in the pharmacy. Even basic pharmacy commodities such as generic nonprescription aspirin products require some level of service. At minimum, someone has to stock the shelf.

The more intangible the offering, the more a business is service-oriented. Businesses whose value lies in the provision of tangible goods, such as manufacturing and retailing, are more product-oriented. Those whose value comes from offering intangible services, such as investment management, consulting, and teaching, are more service-oriented. These service-oriented businesses provide value not in tangible objects but in information, ideas, and processes. Demonstrating the value of intangible offerings requires different strategies than those used for tangible ones. This chapter discusses the characteristics of services.

Service to others is the rent you pay for your room here on earth.

-Muhammad Ali

DEFINING SERVICES

Services can be defined as performances or processes that benefit others. Services can accompany a tangible product or be of value by themselves. Those that accompany a tangible product are often called *value-added services*. They add value by augmenting the value proposition of the tangible product.

Pharmacist services enhance the value proposition of the drug product in a variety of ways. Patient counseling and compliance services increase the effectiveness of drugs. Pharmacist services also make medications more accessible, easier to use, and safer. Value-added pharmacy services include most dispensing activities, automated telephone refill programs, assistance with the selection of nonprescription products, and compounding services.

Some services provide value to consumers without a tangible product. These are called *pure services*. Examples are drug information services, poison information services, patient consultations, and disease-screening activities.

Gronroos[1] groups services into three categories on the basis of their utility (i.e., benefit) to the customer: core services, facilitating services, and supporting services. *Core services* are those that are absolutely essential for the customer to receive a core benefit. A core pharmacist service is one that is necessary to the proper use of medications and to optimal patient outcomes. Filling a prescription for a drug to cure a patient's medical condition might be considered a core service. *Facilitating services* are necessary for the use of core services. Examples in pharmacy are drug inventory control and billing. Without these facilitating services, a needed drug would not be available to dispense. *Supporting services* differ from core and facilitating services in that they are not essential but can increase the value of the core service and differentiate it from the services of competitors. Supporting services depend on the patient's needs; prescription counseling may fall into this category if the patient is already familiar with the drug and is achieving optimal outcomes with it.

LEVELS OF SERVICES

Service performances consist of collections of interactions that can be described on different levels[2] (Figure 7.1).

Service Acts

The smallest unit of service that can be provided is an *act*; a discrete interaction occurring between provider and customer. Acts describe any single point of contact between a business and the people it serves. An example of an act might be a phone call between a pharmacist and a patient or a stop by the customer at the checkout counter. Service acts are also referred to by the alternate terms of *Touchpoints* and *Moments of Truth*.

Acts can happen at any time or place and can be through any marketing channel (e.g., face-to-face, Internet, kiosk). Each act is an opportunity to win or lose a customer. They can be as mundane as a request for directions to the vitamin section of a pharmacy or exceptional like a pharmacist providing CPR to a patient who has collapsed near the prescription department. Acts make up the other service levels of service performance: episodes, experiences, and relationships.

Service Episodes

Service episodes are series of acts over time between the provider and customer. An example of an episode might be a new prescription for an oral antibiotic at a community pharmacy. The process of filling an antibiotic consists of numerous acts or touchpoints between the customer and the pharmacy. The episode might start with a search for the nearest pharmacy on a mobile phone. It may then continue with others acts such as a trip to the pharmacy, a drop off of the prescription, the wait for the medication, and the receipt of the antibiotic along with any counseling. The episode may end with a follow-up call at home by the pharmacist to assess the patient's progress.

Differentiating service acts from episodes can be important in designing complex service systems. Acts are typically completed between a provider (e.g., pharmacist) and customer. Episodes might occur with multiple providers (e.g., pharmacist, technician, and physician) and numerous hand-offs between those providers. Planning service episodes can be done with service scripts. Service scripts delineate the roles and steps in an interaction between provider and customer.[3] Planning for service episodes typically requires mapping service processes with service blueprints[4] or other forms of service mapping.

Figure 7.1 Levels of Service Performance

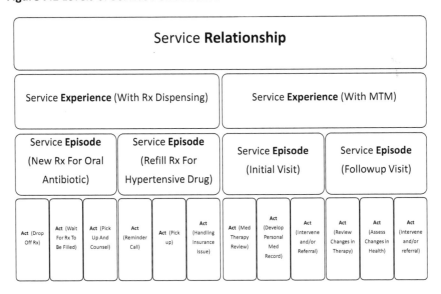

Total Service Experience

A series of episodes provided over time make up the total service experience. A *customer's service experience* is defined as the customer's overall perception of all service episodes received across multiple visits and channels over time.[5] The service experience with a retail pharmacy chain might consist customer perceptions of visits to the pharmacy's website, phone calls to and from the pharmacy, visits to several stores in the chain, and mail order delivery of medications to the customer's home.

Service experiences differ from acts and episodes because they have no specific boundaries with a beginning and end. Each act and episode adds to the overall experience. Particularly good or bad acts or episodes can change a customer's overall perception of a provider's service experience.

Service experiences are often described as a customer's journey through a service system. Marketers often try to understand the customer journey with customer journey maps.[6-8] *Customer journey maps* are diagrams that illustrate the steps customers go through when engaging with a business. Understanding the overall journey helps improve the total experience felt by customers when interacting with a pharmacy. They are a strategic tool that can offer insights into ways to offer service innovations.

Service Relationships

Acts, episodes, and experiences hopefully result in long term relationships between businesses and customers. *Service relationships* are the way in which providers and customers talk to each other, behave in their interactions and engage in the provision of service.[2] Whereas, the service experience is from the customer's point of view, service relationships describe perceptions of the relationship from both the provider and customer perspectives. Relationships are two-way, and strong relationships require commitment by both parties to their roles.[9] This is true in all business relationships, including those in pharmacy.[10, 11]

Service relationships can be described in various ways. Austin and colleagues classify service relationships between pharmacists and patients as existing on a continuum of whether the pharmacist perceives that they are serving a patient, client, customer, or consumer.[12] A pharmacist/patient relationship is one in which the patient is more reliant and the pharmacist more paternalistic in their roles. A pharmacist/client relationship is one where the roles between the two are more emotional and interactive. Pharmacist/customer relationships center on transactions of value, and pharmacist/consumer relationships refer to straight business transactions. The point of this classification is that the acts, episodes, and experiences provided by pharmacies and pharmacists are made up and determined by the relationships pharmacists have with their customers. Pharmacists and patients choose their relationships and the roles they play in them.

CHARACTERISTICS UNIQUE TO SERVICES

When comparing the marketing of services and products, it is clear that services are harder to market. The reason is that services have distinct characteristics that require them to be marketed differently from tangible merchandise such as automobiles and laundry detergent. The ways in which services are unique can be described by the following characteristics (known as the 4I's):

1.   **Intangibility.**   Services are intangible because they are actions and events. They cannot be seen, held, or touched. Thus, their quality cannot be measured, tested, or verified in advance of the sale to ensure excellence.

2.   **Inconsistency.** Services are inconsistent because no two service performances are exactly alike. They vary from person to person, transaction to transaction, and even time to time. Service quality cannot be easily standardized because of the variations among interactions between buyer and seller.

3.   **Inseparability.** The service provider, customers, and service itself are inseparable, because the provider produces the service with the customer's participation. Service quality is determined by both the provider and the customer. In the case of pharmacists' services, patient participation is critical; patients' active role in their therapy is fundamental to medication therapy management. Although the patient may not need to be physically present when a prescription is filled, some patient–provider interaction must occur for the patient to receive the product and use it. Even if the prescription is filled in a distant location by an anonymous pharmacist, there is still a patient–provider interaction when the patient reads the prescription and warning labels provided by the pharmacist. It is with this realization that *patient engagement*, defined as active participation in health care by patients, is becoming an increasingly important issue in health care.[13, 14] The more engaged the patient, the better the resulting outcomes.

4.   **Inventory.** Until recently, most services were mostly provided face-to-face in a real-time, synchronous manner (i.e., person-to-person at a single moment in time). In these situations, services are used as they are being produced, or they are not used at all. Once delivered, synchronous services are lost. Therefore, they cannot be produced prior to their need and put into inventory or on a shelf for later use. However, this characteristic is less relevant in describing services today. Technology now allows us to store many services electronically.

CHALLENGES IN MARKETING SERVICES

"Why does that pharmacist have to be two and a half feet higher than everybody else? Who the hell is this guy? Clear out everybody I'm workin with pills up here. I'm taking pills from this big bottle and then I'm gonna put them in a little bottle! That's my whole job. I can't be down on the floor with you people. Then I'm gonna type out, on a little piece of paper. And it's really hard."

--Jerry Seinfeld (comedian) imitating a pharmacist

Jerry Seinfeld's comedy routines are based upon his observations of the world. In the routine above, he describes how he and a lot of other people see pharmacists -- as taking pills from a big bottle and putting them into a little bottle. Of course, pharmacists know better but it is hard to get the public to see what pharmacist can actually do.

One reason is that pharmacy is a service profession, and the characteristics of services present special challenges in marketing. Some of these challenges are listed in Table 7.1 and discussed in the following sections.

Table 7.1 Challenges in Marketing Services

Characteristic	Challenge
Intangibility	Service quality is difficult for customers to assess
	Services are difficult for marketers to display or describe
	Assigning value and pricing is difficult
Inconsistency	Employee actions determine the quality of services
	Service quality depends on many uncontrollable factors
	The actual service delivered often does not match what was planned and promoted
Inseparability	Customers participate in and influence the service delivered
	Customers influence each others' service experience
Inventory	Many services cannot be stored for later use
	It is hard to synchronize supply and demand with services
	Some services cannot be saved, returned, or resold
	Once some services are delivered, they are lost

Difficult to Promote

Since services cannot be seen, touched, or sensed, it is hard to promote their value to others. It is a challenge for marketers to get customers to notice and desire a product they cannot see or touch. To check this for yourself, try to explain to friends and family members the concept medication therapy management and why it is of value. Then have them describe the concept back to you. The results can be disappointing. The intangible nature of pharmacist services makes it hard for consumers to mentally grasp what pharmacists do. It is much easier for people to grasp the purpose of a drug than to comprehend the pharmacist services associated with that drug.

Hard for Customers to Evaluate

The intangibility of services makes them hard for customers to assess. Although some aspects of services are easy to evaluate (e.g., fast, friendly, inexpensive), other aspects are difficult to evaluate even with extensive experience (e.g., clinical skills). For example, it is unlikely that anyone but a pharmacist would be able to recognize when another pharmacist omits critical drug-related information during patient counseling. In the absence of objective measures of quality, patients use variables that they can assess, such as how a pharmacist looks and acts.

Variable

Another characteristic of services that makes them challenging to assess is their variability. Service providers such as pharmacists are human beings who can be emotional or distracted by constantly changing service conditions. Each service experience can be affected by a host of factors including the work environment (e.g., ringing telephones), the patient (e.g., questions and requests), the pharmacist (e.g., fatigue), and time (e.g., peak commuting time). No one can be certain before visiting a pharmacy what type of service will be experienced.

Often Invisible

Most pharmaceutical services are provided behind the scenes, out of view of the customer. The customer does not see those services and thus cannot appreciate their value unless he or she is made aware of it. Pharmacists who do not inform customers of the "invisible" services they provide get no credit in the eyes of customers for the value they have given.

Supply and Demand Hard to Synchronize

Demand for service is rarely constant in pharmacy settings. Throughout the day and week, there are times when business is relatively slow and other times when it gets quite hectic. It is a problem to synchronize customers' demand for services with the availability of pharmacy personnel to serve them. Synchronizing supply and demand is becoming easier with technology but is still a problem.

The synchronization problem varies by pharmacy setting and type of work provided. In community pharmacies, it is hard to forecast the demand for services at any specific time. Anyone can walk into a pharmacy at any time and ask for service. Although demand can be regulated somewhat through hours of operation and promotional activities, the demand for service is determined largely by the customer. In hospital inpatient settings, the number of patients is limited, so demand is easier to forecast. Many services such as preparation of intravenous admixtures and distribution of maintenance medications can be performed when demand for more immediate services is low.

MARKETING IN ACTION

Branded Service Encounters

Branded service encounters are service interactions where employee behaviors are strategically aligned with the business's brand.[15] This means that employees are the brand, and they are encouraged to speak and act in ways consistent with the brand. Branded service alignment can appear in how an employee greets a customer, the employee's choice of clothing, the eagerness of the employee to help, and any other actions meant to reinforce a customer's perception of a brand.

Zappos online shoe store is an example of a business that uses branded service encounters. Zappos employees support the brand by offering world class services. They are renowned for staying on the phone no matter how long it takes to satisfy a customer. If a caller says she wants to buy a shoe seen the day before on a television show, the Zappos employee will watch the show with the customer if needed to identify the desired shoe. Zappos management encourages this behavior because it is consistent with the company's brand. Zappos.com encourages branded service encounters the following ways.

1. They hire for cultural fit. Zappos chooses employees with a friendly, outgoing personality. This is consistent with one of Zappos' core values to "create fun and a little weirdness." When interviewing potential employees, Zappos managers ask them, "On a scale of one to ten, how weird are you?" Their reaction and response are used to identify applicants' passion, personality, and commitment to customer service.

2. They commit to transparency. Zappos shares everything -- good and bad -- with employees, partners, and vendors. Transparency is important because it shows respect and engenders trust in people.

3. They help employees grow. Everyone at Zappos.com is given the opportunity to interact with a "goal coach" whose job is the help employees identify and meet their personal goals. The idea behind the coach is that if people

achieve their dreams, it makes them happy, and happy employees offer better service.

4. They empower staff to do what's right. Zappos customers are never rushed to make a purchase and to get off the phone. Call center employees have no service scripts or time limits for calls. The primary way of assessing employee success is by asking, "Was the customer happy?" If the answer is consistently yes, employees are rewarded.

5. They deliver happiness, not products. Zappos CEO Tony Hsieh tells people that the company delivers happiness, not shoes. Employees that deliver happiness are promoting the Zappos brand.

Source: Reference[15]

CLASSIFICATION OF PHARMACIST SERVICES

Within the pharmacy profession, services are commonly grouped as shown in Table 7-2: by association with a tangible product, by the type of population being served, or by the setting in which services are provided. Although these classifications are useful, they are insufficient to describe the variety of pharmacy services in the United States. Classifying services associated with a product says little about how the product is provided and ignores instances in which services may accompany no tangible good (e.g., patient education). Describing services by type of population served does not explain how the population is being served. Classifying services according to practice setting makes an implicit assumption that services within each setting are relatively homogeneous; in truth, the levels and types of services provided can vary widely. Pharmacists must look beyond such narrow classifications to recognize innovative ways to serve patients.

Table 7-2 Classification of Pharmacist Services

Services Associated with a Tangible Product

- o Prescription v. Nonprescription medications
- o New prescriptions v. Refills
- o Specialty medicine
- o Unique administration requirements (e.g., IV, IM, transdermal)
- o Complementary and herbal medicine
- o Durable medical equipment
- o Home testing equipment and diagnostics

Services Provided to Specific Populations

- o   Geriatric
- o   Pediatric
- o   Women's health
- o   Disease-specific

Services Associated with a Practice Setting

- o   Hospital: Centralized services v. Decentralized services
- o   Independent v. Chain v. Mass merchandiser v. Grocery store
- o   Mail order or Internet
- o   Long-term care
- o   Home health

Lovelock[16] states that specialization in many service industries has caused inbreeding of ideas and methods. People who work in the hotel, restaurant, and health care industries, for example, tend to remain in these industries for most of their lives. They rely on the same old ways of accomplishing tasks, because they are not exposed to innovative ideas and techniques from other service industries.

Pharmacy is not immune to this inbreeding. Pharmacists and pharmacy managers tend to remain in the profession for most of their lives. Their education and training was provided primarily by pharmacists, so they observe the world primarily through the eyes of a pharmacist. Consequently, they may overlook opportunities that might be readily apparent to people outside the profession.

Pharmacists might benefit from examining their services and products through new eyes. Pharmacist services can be re-categorized according to schemes established by service marketers. By fitting their services into these new classifications, pharmacists can explore how providers in similar service categories address parallel situations.

SERVICE CLASSIFICATIONS FROM THE MARKETING FIELD

Service marketers use other classification systems to analyze services in ways that offer insight into how the services are provided, how the services might be perceived by consumers, and how new strategies for providing services might be identified.[16] Some of these classification systems are presented in this section to stimulate pharmacists to think outside the box when analyzing service marketing opportunities (Table 7-3).

Table 7-3 New ways of Classifying Pharmacist Services

Classification	Variables in Classification
Tangibility of Product/Service Mix	Product or Service Orientation?
Focus of Services	Directed at People or Things?
Need for Customer to be Physically Present	Face-to-Face or Distance Service Delivery?
Need for Customer to be Mentally Present	Engaged or Not Engaged?
Pharmacist/Patient Relationship	Formal or Informal?
Nature of Service Provided	Discrete or Continuous?
Room for Customization and Judgment	Standardized or Customized?
Professionalism of Services	Professional or Non-professional?

Tangibility of the Product–Service Mix

The service mix provided by pharmacists can range from being almost totally product-focused to completely service focused (Figure 7-2). The more product-focused the mix is, the more the pharmacist will adopt strategies consistent with the marketing of tangible goods.[16] The more service-focused the mix is, the more a service strategy is needed.

The left side of Figure 7-2 gives examples of product–service combinations that are more tangible; here, services are less likely to be required in order for the patient to benefit from the product. The right side of the continuum indicates mixes in which intensive services are likely to be needed for the patient to receive a benefit.

The provision of nonprescription (over-the-counter) drugs falls at the left end of the tangibility continuum. Although pharmacists are frequently called upon to assist in the selection of nonprescription drugs, the sale of these products requires few supplemental services beyond delivery and shelf stocking. In fact, nonprescription drugs are common items in vending machines or at gas stations. Home testing kits and other devices require more services, because their use can be more complex than that of nonprescription products. Durable medical equipment, such as crutches and wheelchairs, requires even more service.

Dispensing of medications is found to the right of the center of the continuum. Dispensing of refill medications requires less intensive service than dispensing medications that patients have never used before - additional record keeping, therapeutic review, and patient counseling. Further to the right are medication therapy management services which involve higher levels of personalized care and therapeutic problem solving. Drug information services are at the far right of the continuum because they are all service with no tangible product.

Figure 7.2 Product/Service Orientation

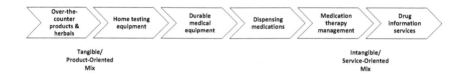

Pharmacists need to decide the degree to which their value proposition is based upon the provision of tangible products or intangible services. The more tangible or product-oriented their value proposition, the more they will adopt strategies consistent with the retailing of merchandise. The more intangible or service-oriented the mix is, the more a service strategy is needed.

Pharmacists will always be associated with tangible drugs because control of medication use is fundamental to the profession. Nevertheless, selling services like MTM and drug information services may require different marketing tactics than traditional retail businesses have used in the past.

Focus of Services

Another way of classifying services is to ask whether they are directed at people or things.[16] Pharmacy services can be classified as (1) tangible actions to people's bodies, such as vaccinations and disease screening; (2) tangible actions to things, such as retail dispensing, veterinary pharmacy, and mail order; (3) intangible actions directed at people, such as patient education and drug information services; or (4) intangible actions directed at intangible assets, such as pharmacy benefit design and drug-use review (Table 7-4).

This categorization is useful because it forces pharmacists to answer some important questions about their services:

1. Does the patient need to be physically present to receive the service? If one considers pharmacist services to consist of tangible actions directed at goods, then the answer is probably no. Pharmacists can provide basic dispensing services at a distant location and send the drugs by courier or mail. However, services such as vaccination and cholesterol screening require the presence of the patient.

2. Does the patient need to be mentally present during the service process? Intensive counseling sessions require patients to be present, ready, and engaged. If the patient is distracted or fatigued, much of the benefit of counseling will be lost.

Table 7-4 Pharmacist Services Classified by the Nature of the Service Act

Action Type	Directed at People	Directed at Things
Tangible	Services directed at people's bodies - Vaccinations - Blood pressure monitoring - Cholesterol testing - Diabetes screening	Services directed at goods and other physical possessions - Drug dispensing - OTC counseling - Durable medical equipment - Herbal medicines - Veterinary medicine - Mail order pharmacy
Intangible	Services directed at people's minds - Patient education - Drug information services - Alternative medicine	Services directed at intangible assets - Drug insurance design - Pharmacy benefit management - Drug-use review

Type of Customer Relationship

Pharmacists' services can be classified by the type of relationship with the patient. Relationships can be defined according to (1) whether there is a formal relationship between patient and provider and (2) whether services are provided on a continual basis over time or as discrete transactions.

Many patients have no formal relationship with their pharmacies. Anyone with a prescription can walk into most community pharmacies for service. However, formal relationships are becoming more common. With the advent of drug insurance, customers of prescription drug services often enter into contracts to use network pharmacies. In these relationships, membership is usually with the drug insurance plan, not the pharmacy. In other cases, pharmacy providers develop direct, formal relationships with their customers through loyalty card programs. In loyalty card programs, patients show their card when purchasing merchandise to receive a discount or other benefit. In return, the pharmacy can gather information on patients' purchasing habits and provide incentives to continue patronizing the pharmacy.

Whether pharmacists provide continual or discrete services depends on patient needs and preferences and provider business strategies. If a patient needs to visit a pharmacy only for occasional acute conditions such as a minor skin rash, continual services may be unnecessary. Or, the consumer may prefer to shop at several different pharmacies, depending on price, convenience, or variety. For this consumer, variety and low prices may be more important than continuity. Furthermore, some pharmacies use a high-volume, low-price business strategy that by its very nature can discourage continuity of services. In order to maintain high volume and low prices, patient–pharmacist interactions need to be kept to a minimum, so there is little opportunity to develop a personal relationship. Other pharmacies emphasize a service mix targeted toward patients who desire and need personalized, ongoing care. These providers seek strong bonds with patients who can be served profitably over time.

Room for Customization and Judgment

The role of customization and judgment in the practice of pharmacy has changed over the years. In the past, pharmacists were responsible for compounding most of the drugs provided for customers. They would mix different combinations of medications individualized to each patient's medical condition. Compounding was unique to the pharmacy profession and one of the things that distinguished pharmacists from all other professionals.

Now, pharmacists rarely compound medications in typical practice. Most of the drugs dispensed are purchased from pharmaceutical manufacturers in standardized forms and doses, often in unit-of-use packages (i.e., ready to be dispensed after application of a prescription label). In current practice, most customization by pharmacists comes in the provision of services.

All services can be classified by their potential for customization and judgment. Many services are standardized and do not easily permit customization. For example, people expect that when they enter a movie theater, services will be provided in a set sequence: pay for the ticket, give it to the ticket taker, buy refreshments, find a seat, and see the movie at the scheduled time. Both the service provider and the customer follow this sequence of steps. Most movie theaters serve the same selection of refreshments: popcorn, soft drinks, and candy. This is expected. It is also expected that movie patrons will wait in line, scan the concession menu above the snack bar, and make a choice quickly and without much deviation from the menu.

The provider and customer are expected to act in ways consistent with their roles. If the movie theater makes a substitution for any concession snack item (e.g., fresh vegetables for popcorn), movie patrons may get upset. On the other hand, theater employees will become impatient if a patron orders snack items that are not on the menu. The expectations of both customers and providers discourage the performance of services outside those expectations. Standardized sequences of events occur with mass merchandise retailers, public transportation, quick-oil-change businesses, and many other services.

The potential for customization also depends on the degree to which frontline service personnel can exercise judgment in meeting the needs of customers. In standardized service situations, the responsibilities and roles of customer contact personnel are restricted. A cook in a fast food restaurant is not allowed to provide items that are not on the menu, a bus driver cannot take new routes to a destination, and a quick-oil-change mechanic cannot fix mufflers. In other words, the nature of individual jobs can limit customization.

Jobs such as those in the legal and health care professions cannot be easily standardized. Although some standardization can occur in medicine (e.g., urgent care centers) and law (e.g., standardized wills), many of the problems seen in these professions are too complex for standardized solutions. For instance, problems in surgery and radiation oncology are likely to require solutions that take into account numerous unpredictable factors. Other areas in which standardization is difficult include architecture, home repair, and real estate.

In most businesses the choice between customization and standardization is a strategic decision. Customization can differentiate one business from another and establish a competitive advantage. Customized service can often provide an advantage because it is tailored to the specific needs of customers, but customization can be more expensive because it requires greater personnel time and financial resources. Standardization can lower costs by increasing efficiency so that fewer personnel are needed to serve customers. This can permit businesses to offer lower prices without reducing profitability.

Professional and Nonprofessional Services

Services can be classified as professional or nonprofessional. Professional services are provided by individuals who are members of a profession, such as physicians, lawyers, and pharmacists. Professionals are distinguished from nonprofessionals by the following characteristics:[17]

- o Professionals are considered to have unique skills, expertise, and training that nonprofessionals do not.

- o Professionals have a distinct group identity and are largely self-regulating.

- o Professionals are experts in specialized fields and use their expertise to advise and assist customers in solving problems.

Professional services are distinct from nonprofessional services in several ways.[17] Professional services are more complex and require more extensive problem-solving skills and expertise. Consumer perceptions of risk are greater with professional services, because of the complexity of problems dealt with by professionals. In addition, consumers perceive themselves to be less able to assess the quality of professional services because of insufficient expertise and training.

Being perceived as a professional has several strategic implications for pharmacists.[17] Consumers tend to perceive professional services as important and are inclined to be less sensitive to the pricing of these services. When professional issues such as health or financial well-being are at stake, consumers are less likely to pinch pennies. Also, perceptions of expertise are more important in selecting professional services. Consumers place greater weight on the technical expertise of professionals because it is this expertise that determines a successful outcome. Finally, word-of-mouth recommendations are more important in marketing communications for professional services than are advertising and other paid forms of promotion. Since professional services are perceived to involve more risk, consumers gravitate toward more credible sources of product and service information, such as recommendations from friends and family.

MEETING THE CHALLENGES IN PROVIDING SERVICES

Tangible Clues to Quality

When customers have difficulty evaluating pharmaceutical services because of intangibility, they look for tangible clues to quality.

Tangible clues are things such as the lighting, cleanliness, and neatness of a pharmacy practice site. Other tangible clues can include the dress, appearance, and body language of the pharmacist; the manner in which merchandise is organized on the shelves; and the quality of patient information leaflets. Pharmacists who want to project an image of quality must pay attention to these details.

MARKETING IN ACTION

Looks Really Do Count

Exceptional pharmacist services and low prices won't do much for your business if customers are turned off by the looks of your pharmacy and employees. First and second impressions count when people visit pharmacies. Bad signage on the outside and inside of a pharmacy, messy aisles, dirty facilities, and sloppily dressed employees can make a customer's first impression the only one because they never return. To illustrate with a personal story:

"I took my wife Diane to a local Thai restaurant. We were looking forward to the meal because we heard good things about it on Yelp. Our excitement turned to revulsion when we grabbed the handle of the restaurant door. Looking at us through the glass restaurant door was a big cockroach! We immediately turned around and never returned. Now it is possible that this was a one-time event and that the restaurant is perfectly clean and well run. But we will never know because our negative first impression of the restaurant is burned into our memory."

Marketers call the physical environment seen and felt by customers the "servicescape."[18] The servicescape describes the environment in which the service is assembled and where the service experience occurs. For a community pharmacy, it includes the stores exterior appearance (parking, exterior design, landscaping, signage, and neighborhood) and interior environment (merchandising, signage, store layout, decor, colors, sounds, smells, temperature, and overall ambiance).

Pharmacists need to know that they can lose customers before they ever enter a pharmacy. Taking a store's external appearance for granted with poor signage and messy parking lots can lose customers to competing pharmacies who are more meticulous. Once inside the pharmacy, the quality of the internal appearance needs to be equally inviting to move them throughout the store. Any detail that is ignored from musical choice to aisle width to lighting can determine how much is purchased and how long a patron lingers in the store.

Tangible Evidence of Service

When providing pure services with no tangible product, give people something they can feel and touch as evidence that they have received something of value. When educating patients, give them something in writing, such as a patient package insert or a written care plan, to remind them of what was discussed. In addition to the value provided by the information on the insert or plan, patients then have something to remind them that a valuable transaction took place.

Word-of-Mouth Promotion

The more complex the service, the more likely it is that consumers will use word-of-mouth recommendations from friends, acquaintances, and family members in choosing pharmacists and pharmacies. As personal sources of recommendation become more important, pharmacists should attempt to tap into this trend by encouraging customer "word-of-mouth."

There are several strategies pharmacists can use to increase word-of-mouth communication. The first is to ask customers to recommend the pharmacy to others. The request can be simple: "If you are happy with our service, please recommend us to family or friends." As relationships with customers strengthen, pharmacists should look for opportunities to subtly encourage recommendations. The pharmacist might say, "John, I haven't seen your wife in here lately. Has she been taking her blood pressure medicine consistently?"

Professionalism

Although pharmacy is a profession, not all pharmacists are recognized as professionals by customers. The image of individual pharmacists is determined by how they interact daily with their customers. Pharmacists who consistently demonstrate good decisions, judgment, and professionalism are likely be perceived as professionals. Pharmacists who do not demonstrate their expertise, are unprofessional in their interactions with customers, and minimize patient contact are less likely to be perceived as professionals.

Pharmacists should promote the professional nature of their services. Promotional communications should emphasize pharmacists' expertise, competence, and training. Pharmacists should never pass up an opportunity to teach patients about how they ensure patient safety and positive health outcomes. When a pharmacist identifies a drug-related problem, he should explain to the patient the nature of the problem and the actions he will be taking to resolve it. If every pharmacist did this on a daily basis, people would be more likely to characterize pharmacists as professionals.

Strong Positive Image of the Business

When consumers lack the information or ability to judge the quality of a business, they often rely on general perceptions in choosing where to do business. Impressions about quality are more important when businesses offer products that might be perceived as risky.

Many businesses attempt to establish a strong image of their firm in the minds of customers. A well-known and respected image can reduce customers' perception of risk. Think of the names Google, Geico, Mercedes-Benz, and Pfizer. Each evokes a strong image of quality that makes the business stand out from competitors. Similarly, excellent pharmacies and pharmacists can establish and maintain a strong positive image through promotional communications and other elements of the marketing mix.

Relationship Marketing

Pharmacists should target patients who want or need to establish and maintain long-term formal and informal relationships with pharmacists. Pharmacists can benefit in several ways. With formal membership relationships, it is much easier to collect data reflecting the needs and wants of patients. Patients who use loyalty cards or participate in a managed care plan provide identification that can be used to understand purchasing habits. With that information, services can be customized to specific patient needs. Also, membership pricing can be implemented with formal relationships. A single membership fee can be charged for patients who enroll in a disease management or wellness clinic. One price is charged for the bundle of services, rather than separate prices charged a la carte for medication review, physical assessment, counseling, and various other services provided in a program. Finally, patients who maintain long-term formal or informal relationships are cheaper and more profitable to serve. Loyal patients tend to spend more money and be less price-sensitive than other consumers, and they require the same level of advertising and promotion.[19]

SUMMARY

Most successful businesses attempt to emulate the best practices of all businesses, not just those within their own narrow field. Health care providers now realize that they can learn a lot from the best practices of a variety of service-oriented businesses, including the hospitality, retailing, and food service industries. One of the main goals of this chapter has been to convey the message that the pharmacy profession needs to look beyond its current practices and explore how other businesses serve customers.

Reference List

(1) Gronroos C. Service Marketing and Management. Lexington, MA.: Lexington Books; 1990.

(2) Chandler JD, Lusch RF. Service Systems A Broadened Framework and Research Agenda on Value Propositions, Engagement, and Service Experience. Journal of Service Research 2014;1094670514537709.

(3) Holdford D. Service scripts: a tool for teaching pharmacy students how to handle common practice situations. Am J Pharm Educ 2006;70(1):2.

(4) Holdford DA, Kennedy DT. Service blueprint as a tool for designing innovative pharmaceutical services. Journal of the American Pharmaceutical Association 39[Jul-Aug], 545-552. 1999.

(5) Rawson A, Duncan E, Jones C. The truth about customer experience. Harvard Business Review 2013;91(9):90-98.

(6) David WN, Pine II BJ. Using the customer journey to road test and refine the business model. Strategy & Leadership 2013;41(2):12-17.

(7) Court D, Elzinga D, Mulder S, Vetvik OJ. The consumer journey. McKinsey Quarterly [June]. 2009.

(8) Robert J, Xiangyu K. The customer experience: a road-map for improvement. Managing Service Quality 2011;21(1):5-24.

(9) Morgan RM, Hunt SD. The commitment-trust theory of relationship marketing. the journal of marketing 1994;20-38.

(10) Worley MM, Schommer JC, Brown LM et al. Pharmacists' and patients' roles in the pharmacist-patient relationship: are pharmacists and patients reading from the same relationship script? Res Social Adm Pharm 2007;3(1):47-69.

(11) Maniscalco C, Daniloski K, Brinberg D. The Impact of Relationship Stage on the Determinants of Trust in the Pharmacist–ÇôClient Relationship: Results from a Social Marketing Campaign. Social Marketing Quarterly 2010;16(4):18-40.

(12) Austin Z, Gregory PA, Martin JC. Characterizing the professional relationships of community pharmacists. Research in Social and Administrative Pharmacy 2006;2(4):533-546.

(13) Gerber LM, Barron Y, Mongoven J et al. Activation among chronically ill older adults with complex medical needs: challenges to supporting effective self-management. J Ambul Care Manage 2011;34(3):292-303.

(14) Hibbard JH, Greene J. What the evidence shows about patient activation: better health outcomes and care experiences; fewer data on costs. Health Aff (Millwood) 2013;32(2):207-214.

(15) Sirianni NJ, Bitner MJ, Brown SW, Mandel N. Branded service encounters: Strategically aligning employee behavior with the brand positioning. Journal of Marketing 2013;77(6):108-123.

(16) Lovelock CH. Classifying services to gain strategic marketing insights. Journal of Marketing 1983;47:9-20.

(17) Jeanne Hill C. Differences in the consumer decision process for professional vs. generic services. Journal of Services Marketing 1988;2(1):17-23.

(18) Bitner MJ. Servicescapes: the impact of physical surroundings on customers and employees. Journal of Marketing 1992;56(April):57-61.

(19) Zeithaml VA, MJ. B. Services Marketing. 1st ed. New York: McGraw-Hill Companies Inc.; 1996.

Chapter Questions

1. Does the average pharmacy in your community emphasize product-oriented or service-oriented marketing strategies? Explain the reason for your answer.

2. Which is better for patients: customized or standardized pharmaceutical services? Explain.

3. Provide arguments for why pharmacist services should be classified as "professional."

Activity

We all have service encounters every week with restaurants, bars, banks, airlines, gas stations, dry cleaners, hair stylists, physicians, libraries, schools, car repair shops, copy centers, and others. Record 10 "journal" entries describing service encounters that you experience in the next week. Attempt to include a variety of service businesses and types (e.g., services provided by automation, over the telephone, by Internet, in person). Include satisfying and dissatisfying encounters. Record factual information (when, where, nature of service encounter), your expectations prior to the encounter, a description of the service delivery process, your assessment of its quality (on a scale from 1 to 10), and your perceptions and feelings about each service experience. Note any concepts from this book that are pertinent to your service experience. It is essential that you complete the journal entries on the day of the service and not rely on your memory to recreate them later. Finally, write a one-page report on what you learned from this experience.

CHAPTER **8**

MANAGING SERVICE PERFORMANCE

Objectives

After studying this chapter, the reader should be able to

- List some causes of poor pharmacy service
- Discuss what elements are necessary for a pharmacy to provide good customer service
- Describe the characteristics of good service employees
- Justify the link between internal marketing and business profitability
- Define the following terms: customer-oriented culture, service–profit cycle
- Design a continuous quality improvement plan for pharmacist services

Pharmacy practice places tremendous emphasis on service to customers. Competition for patients is fierce, and service differentiates one pharmacy from the next. The drugs in any pharmacy are essentially the same, but the service is not. The prescription drug received from a Walgreens store is no different from the one filled at CVS. It is the service provided with the drug that varies from pharmacy to pharmacy.

Service can differ in terms of accessibility, merchandise display, technical quality, friendliness, helpfulness, and many other dimensions. Service, along with price, determines the success of a pharmacy in gaining and keeping patients.

Not all pharmacies provide good service. I have seen the following examples of poor service in pharmacies:

- A pharmacist made his coworkers laugh when he regaled them with a story about "telling off" a patient.

- Irritated by the incessant ringing of a telephone, a pharmacist picked up the receiver and slammed it back down without answering.

- When a patient complained that the price of a drug is too high, the pharmacist flippantly responded, "You can always go to the pharmacy down the street." A nearby pharmacy student nodded his head in agreement.

Situations like these, in which pharmacists gave poor service to patients, are not uncommon. Most pharmacy students, pharmacists, and technicians can cite similar anecdotes about poor service. Often they confess that they too have provided poor service at times.

Poor service is not just rude or discourteous behavior. It is failure of pharmacists to meet their professional responsibilities. Pharmacists who fail in their professional obligations can cause avoidable deaths and other negative health outcomes.

When poor service occurs, it may be because the pharmacist is under stress or some circumstance causes him or her to act in an uncharacteristic way. Patients may have been especially demanding or rude. The pharmacist may have been working all day without a break and simply reacted badly due to fatigue and hunger. He or she may have been working without much support from co-workers and management. The stress of the job may have chipped away at the pharmacist's self control, leading him or her to act unprofessionally.

But no matter the reason, poor pharmacy service is unacceptable. It cannot be tolerated—by pharmacists, patients, payers, or pharmacy managers. At the very least, poor pharmacy service can cause patients to take their business elsewhere.

At worst, poor service can cause patient injury or death. Pharmacists who discourage requests for counseling or cut corners by not checking medication profiles can physically harm the people who rely on their professional expertise and behavior. Pharmacists and other health care professionals cannot be permitted the luxury of providing bad service. One lapse in service delivery can destroy years spent building a good patient relationship. It can even end a pharmacist's career or a patient's life.

DIFFICULTIES WITH SERVING PATIENTS

Health care differs from non-health care service in many ways.[1] Pharmacists must serve a variety of needs ranging from the mundane (filling a prescription) to the critical (responding to a code in a hospital). Pharmacists need to tend to physical and emotional requirements of patients under circumstances that might be hectic and less than ideal. Health care services are complicated because:[1]

o *Customers are sick.* Patients who are sick, uncertain, fearful, in pain, and stressed can be difficult to serve. Pharmacists need to be tolerant and compassionate, responding respectfully and professionally to patients.

o *Customers are reluctant.* Illnesses force patients to do things they do not want or are not trained to do. And even worse, they are asked to pay for those things. Pharmacists must overcome that reluctance to serve these patients.

o *Customers are at risk.* Health care is unsafe to customers compared to most other services. Thousands of people are harmed each year through errors and missed opportunities when receiving health and pharmaceutical care.[2] Pharmacists who fail to provide patient centric care put patients at even greater risk. Poor communication, listening, monitoring, and record keeping can lead to errors in prescribing, dispensing, and taking medicines.

CAUSES OF POOR PHARMACY SERVICE

Some pharmacists do not realize they are providing poor service. A young pharmacist who rudely tells the patient, "If you don't like our service, you can go down the street" may not see it as unprofessional behavior. This response might have just been learned by observing co-workers, even supervisors.

In other situations, they are just frustrated and have lost control. Although we may all feel like expressing our frustrations this way from time to time, as professionals we must learn to control our impulses.

Poor service can also result when a pharmacist is the "wrong fit" for a service job. Not everyone is interested in or suited for working with patients.

On the other hand, some pharmacists who have the potential to provide good service simply have not developed the skills and habits to do so. They may lack sufficient communication and counseling skills or have poor work habits that lead to inefficiency and inattention to detail.

In many cases, poor service is not the fault of the pharmacist but of the system in which the pharmacist works. Poor service can be built into a system through poor design, management, recruitment, retention, and training. For example, failure to screen for drug interactions can have a variety of causes, including computer systems that incorrectly identify potential drug interactions as needing attention, pharmacists who have unclear policies for dealing with drug interactions, and managers who emphasize prescription volume over patient safety. These system problems contribute to poor pharmacist performance.

Providing good customer service is not easy. If it were easy, people would never have their prescriptions mixed up in a pharmacy, wait long periods on the telephone or in checkout lines, or be subjected to rude or incompetent service workers.

In the practice of pharmacy, it is particularly difficult to provide good service. Pharmacists are not simply required to provide fast and friendly service. They must maintain accurate patient records, monitor therapy, communicate with and educate patients, and watch out for the patient's welfare.

Every job is a self-portrait of the person who did it.
Autograph your work with excellence.

— *Anonymous*

ELEMENTS OF GOOD CUSTOMER SERVICE

Good customer service depends on several important factors.[3-5] First, it requires the support of a customer-oriented organization—one that emphasizes service leadership, investment in employee training and development, and teamwork. The second key factor is selection and retention of good employees, who are needed to provide good service. Third, good customer service depends on a well-designed and well-run service system. This chapter discusses each of these factors.

Customer-Oriented Organizational Culture

In a customer-oriented organizational culture, everyone recognizes that the organization exists for one reason: to serve the customer.[6,7] People in customer-oriented organizations know that without the customer, there would be no organization. The customer determines the success or failure of the firm. Customer orientation requires that everyone, from the chief executive officer to the service line employee, be devoted to meeting customer needs and wants. This includes the practice of pharmacy.[8,9]

Defining customer orientation can be difficult to do. It is best described by a culture where each employee can truthfully make the following statements:

1. I always go out of my way to assist my customers.
2. I am never too busy to help coworkers and customers.
3. I always persuade customers rather than pressure them.
4. I continually assess my customers' needs.
5. I am willing to disagree with customers to help them make better decisions.
6. I never put my personal needs before the customers'.
7. I continually look for opportunities to help my coworkers and customers.
8. I never pretend that I cannot help customers and coworkers when I really can.
9. I never ignore customers when I am busy.
10. I can always control my emotions when dealing with customers and coworkers.

MARKETING IN ACTION

Is the Customer Always Right?

It is commonly said in business that "the customer is always right". But does this adage really offer the best advice for serving customers? What cases can be made for and against the customer always being right?

The Case For the Customer Always Being Right

1. Without the customer, there is no business. Customers are needed to generate revenue and keep the company in business. Of course, some customers make unreasonable demands and can be disrespectful of the people who serve them. But happy customers are the key to business success.

2. It is easier and cheaper to keep current customers than attract new ones. Attracting new customers requires expensive advertising, coupons, and other promotional strategies. In contrast, it costs less time and effort to keep existing customers happy by going the extra mile to show them you care for them and their business. Great customer service also generates additional business through positive word-of-mouth recommendations and referrals.

3. Negative comments from customers about bad service can spread like a virus. Even if the customer is truly wrong, dissatisfied customers can poison the business's public image with negative web posts and verbal complaints to friends and family members. It is better to give them what they want than to deal with the consequences of their dissatisfaction.

The Case Against the Customer Always Being Right

1. Sometimes what the customer wants can be harmful to their health. This is especially true in pharmacy practice where abuse of medications like antibiotics and controlled substance can hurt people.

2. Sometimes what the customer wants is illegal or unethical. Pharmacists take an oath that delineates their professional responsibilities. Sometimes fulfilling that oath may dissatisfy the customer. This does not mean that the oath or legal restraints should be used as an excuse for not serving the patient. Rather, it means that pharmacists have ethical and legal responsibilities that may be contrary to the customer always being right.

3. Customers are often poor judges of what they need or want. Sometimes a pharmacist has to say "No" along the path to finding the best solution. Often, the best solution results when a pharmacist advocates for a customer's initial desire. Sometimes a pharmacist has to engage in productive conflict to achieve the best outcome.

4. Blind obedience to the rule is disrespectful to employees and can make them resentful. Managers who back customers who are abusive, disrespectful, threatening, or bullies over their loyal, hard-working employees will lose employee trust and commitment to the job.

Therefore, it seems that a case can be made for and against the maxim that the employee is always right. A better maxim might be, "The customer should always feel that a business and its employees do everything they can to serve the customer's needs."

This new rule puts the customer first, but does not make unreasonable demands of employees. With this rule, employees are given permission to say "no" but only in limited situations. Employees also need to be trained to say "no" in a way that respects and appreciates the customer and communicates a desire to help. Employees can substitute the word "no" with probing questions, suggest alternative solutions, or just acknowledge the customer's request. Proper employee training in how to say "No" can establish high expectations for employee efforts without making them feeling disrespected by management.

Service Leadership

Customer orientation in any pharmacy organization starts at the top.[10,11] The pharmacy leader sets the organization's direction and priorities. If service is not foremost in the mind of pharmacy leaders, it will not be a priority at the pharmacy staff level.

Good service organizations have strong leaders who stress the importance of service in both words and actions. They are committed to service and are able to communicate their commitment to service to others within the organization.

Leadership was key to the excellent service offered at Ukrops, a beloved family owned grocery chain in Richmond, Virginia that has since been purchased by the Martins grocery chain. All newly hired Ukrop employees were oriented by the company's president, Bobby Ukrop, to the company's values and its commitment to the community. The vision of extraordinary customer service was delivered to everyone including managers, pharmacists, baggers, cashiers, and stockers. Company values were continually reinforced and modeled by everyone throughout the company. Locals still talk about how much they miss Ukrops and its exceptional service.

Service leadership can occur at many levels. It can be shown by the independent pharmacy owner, the hospital pharmacy director, the chief executive officer of a national pharmacy chain, and even the pharmacist in charge at a community pharmacy. The higher up in an organization that commitment to service exists; the more likely it will be an organization wide priority.

The leader's role in communicating a coherent vision to subordinates cannot be underestimated. A shared vision of service can excite people and motivate them toward common goals.

President John F. Kennedy illustrated the power of vision when he told the world, in the 1960s, that America would have a man on the moon by the end of the decade. At the time, travel to the moon seemed impossible. Nevertheless, President Kennedy's vision helped energize the American people to support the efforts of the U.S. space program. This compelling vision led the United States to put a man on the moon in 1969, after Kennedy's death.

Pharmacy service organizations can benefit from inspirational leadership. The practice of pharmacy is no less important than going to the moon. People put their trust and their health in the hands of pharmacists, and pharmacists should realize that what they do is more than just a job. Practicing pharmacy is too difficult without the feeling that it has some meaning or value. Good leaders can provide pharmacy employees with an inspirational vision of the organization and the profession.

Investment in Training and Development

Excellent pharmacies invest in the training and development of their employees.[5, 12] This involves more than just paying pharmacists to attend continuing-education programs to meet state licensing requirements. It means providing job-based training that can help pharmacists to do their jobs better and to progress in their careers.

Pharmacists in service organizations cannot be expected to perform well if they lack the appropriate skills and knowledge to do their jobs correctly. Pharmacists need training and development throughout their careers. Even pharmacists with extensive practice experience need to periodically renew their skills to keep up with changes in the profession.

In addition to updating employees' knowledge, training and development can help build confidence, enhance intrinsic motivation, and promote self-esteem.[5] Often, employees know what to do but lack the confidence to do it. Proper training can also enhance service by making job tasks more interesting and fulfilling. The more people know about their jobs, the more they can become involved in the details and delivery. A repetitive task, such as filling a prescription, is much more interesting if the pharmacist understands the therapeutics of the drug being dispensed, the diseases suffered by the patient, and the methods and theories of patient counseling. The more the pharmacist knows, the more he or she is enriched by the job.

Systematic training is planned and scheduled, and the training methods are based on the needs of the individual and the organization. Some skills might be learned from another employee, others might be developed through a continuing-education program offered by a pharmacy association, and others might be learned on the job through trial and error. The key is that it helps pharmacists and other employees serve customers better.

Teamwork

The practice of pharmacy can be demanding and stressful without the support of coworkers. Pharmacists often have heavy workloads that may prevent them from practicing pharmacy the way they would like to without assistance. A community pharmacist may have one patient who requires extensive counseling about a medication, another who wants to discuss why his insurance company will not pay for his medication, a third who has a potential drug interaction, and three more patients who need their prescriptions filled. Under these conditions, it may be impossible to satisfy everyone without working as part of a team.

Teamwork can help pharmacists deal with the demands of their jobs. Knowing that other pharmacists and technicians are available and willing to help can reduce stress when things get busy. In addition to helping with the physical work, co-workers can offer moral support. For instance, a pharmacist who has just been criticized by a physician or patient may be quite upset. Co-workers can help by simply listening while the pharmacist vents frustrations and concerns.

Co-workers can also share successful solutions to problems. In some pharmacies, unusual or difficult problems are electronically posted in a way that is readily available to all employees. An employee documents a problem in a post, the circumstances behind the difficulty, and how it was solved. Other employees are expected to read the posts periodically so they can benefit from the experiences of others. Another way of sharing is to hold periodic meetings to discuss interesting patient cases. One pharmacist describes a difficult patient case and how he or she dealt with it, and learning takes place through group discussion.

Often, pharmacists work with nonpharmacist professionals on inter-professional teams. A specific problem (e.g., how do we reduce medication errors?) may be identified and addressed in team meetings. Since many problems and solutions in pharmacy practice originate outside the pharmacy, participation on interprofessional teams is important.

Selecting and Keeping Good Employees

Quality service is built through the selection and retention of quality workers. Employers compete for talented pharmacy employees, not just to fill open positions but to keep good employees from leaving to work for competitors.

Excellent service organizations try hard to recruit excellent workers. The best service workers have not only good skills and intelligence, but the right attitude. Employers select and keep service employees who have a good balance of knowledge, skills, and attitude.

Internal Marketing

Employers need to market themselves to attract and keep talented employees; this is *internal marketing*.[13] Employers have a product (i.e., a job) that needs to be marketed to customers (i.e., potential and current employees). Components of the product might include a good work environment, acceptable pay and benefits, and the opportunity to learn and progress within the job.

Employers can aggressively market to potential and existing employees. In internal marketing, management treats employees the same way external customers are treated. Employers conduct market research to identify employee needs (e.g., through employee satisfaction surveys), develop an attractive product offering (e.g., salary, challenging work), and promote that offering through different forms of marketing communications (e.g., want ads, word of mouth).

The more desirable the job, the better management is able to select the best employees to serve customers. An employer who has and markets the best jobs becomes the employer of choice for employees. Employers of choice have fewer problems with job turnover, because employees do not want to leave. When vacancies occur, they are filled quickly. In many cases, want ads are unnecessary; word-of-mouth recommendations from current employees result in a sufficient number of applicants.

The relationships among internal marketing, customer service, and profitability of the firm can be envisioned as a continuous cycle.[14,15] Treating employees well leads to employee satisfaction and retention. Satisfied employees are more likely to appreciate their jobs and have the attitude necessary to provide good service. Happy employees project that happiness to customers and are more enjoyable to be around. Customers are more satisfied and likely to be loyal. Loyal customers generate greater revenue and greater profit for the firm.

The development of an internal marketing environment involves the following steps:[16]

- o Educating employees about the internal marketing concept and the existence of internal customers.

- o Having employees and managers identify their internal customers.

- o Helping employees and managers identify the expectations of their internal customers.

- o Developing strategies to meet the needs of internal customers, such as providing opportunities for professional development and job enrichment for subordinates.

- o Monitoring internal customer satisfaction and other benchmark measures (e.g., customer satisfaction surveys, exit interviews, employee telephone hotlines, suggestion boxes).

Employee Recruitment

Excellent service employers never stop searching for employees. Even when no positions are open, they keep a list of potential employees whom they can contact when an opening occurs. They proactively develop a pool of qualified candidates through work contacts and networking at professional meetings. Current employees also help by recommending the company to potential candidates and contacting them when a position opens. Proactive recruitment is useful because little time is lost when employees leave. When an opening occurs, qualified candidates are interviewed and hired as quickly as possible in order to maintain continuity of service. This puts them two steps ahead of reactive organizations that only start recruiting when a job opening occurs.

Employee Retention

Keeping good employees is one of the biggest challenges faced by pharmacist employers. The loss of key employees can have a devastating effect on pharmacies. In one neighborhood in Virginia, people still talk about "Billy," a pharmacist at a pharmacy chain store. Billy lived in the neighborhood of the pharmacy, and many people who visited the pharmacy were his friends. Billy often came from behind the pharmacy counter to talk to patients about their therapy and lives. Billy knew all of his customers by name, and after he left, the store was never the same. Temporary pharmacists rotated in and out. Patients lost their sense of loyalty to the store and started going to nearby competitors. Even years after Billy's departure, patients complained that they missed the relationship they'd had when he was their pharmacist.

Pharmacists build bonds of trust with their patients, and those bonds are extended to the pharmacy. When a key pharmacist leaves, the bond to both the employee and the pharmacy is broken. A new pharmacist has to rebuild the bond, and that can take time.

The cost of losing a pharmacist can be high. In institutional practice, the costs of turnover has been estimated to range from more than 20 thousand dollars to almost 90 thousand dollars per pharmacist.[17]

In addition to the costs for recruitment, selection, and training; the firm might suffer lost managerial time, reduced efficiency, productivity losses, and lost business associated with new employees. The loss of a pharmacist can cause multiple problems:

o The pharmacy may have to reduce store hours until a replacement can be found.

o Patients may go to competitors.

o The remaining pharmacists and employees have to cover the responsibilities of the missing pharmacist. This can increase employee stress and lead to more overtime costs to the pharmacy.

o The employer incurs costs to replace the pharmacist. The employer may pay to advertise the position in newspaper want ads or professional journals. Current personnel must be paid for performing related clerical and interviewing tasks.

o Personnel need to be freed from their usual responsibilities so they can train newly hired pharmacists.

o A new pharmacist may take a year or more to become 100% productive. Productivity is reduced while the pharmacist learns job details such as the location of drugs, computer system procedures, and proper handling of insurance forms.

Employers need to invest as much in keeping employees as they do in recruiting them. Adopting an internal marketing philosophy is a good start. In pharmacy practice, excellent service comes down to finding and keeping excellent workers. Without excellent employees, it is much more difficult to succeed in marketing.

Well-Designed and Well-Run Service Systems

Even the best employees have difficulty providing good service in service settings that are poorly designed and run. In many businesses, poor service is designed into the system, as illustrated in the following scenarios.

Scenario 1: At 8:55 am, a hospital nurse goes to the medication room to get a 9 am medication for a patient but finds no drug in the patient's cassette. Knowing how much work she has to do, the nurse tries to save time by checking the medication cassettes of other patients for an extra dose that she can "borrow." Having no luck, she telephones the pharmacy. A pharmacist answers after the 15th ring. The nurse asks the pharmacist to send the missing medication to the nursing unit as soon as possible. The pharmacist checks the patient's computer record to see if an order has been received for the medication. Finding no record of the order in the computer, the pharmacist asks the nurse to see if the order has been sent to the pharmacy yet. Exasperated, the nurse hangs up the phone and searches for the order on the nursing unit. She quickly finds that the order has not yet been picked up by the hospital courier. Knowing that the patient needs the dose before a scheduled X-ray procedure at 10 am, the nurse goes to the central pharmacy to have the medication order filled. At the central pharmacy, she has to wait for 5 minutes while the pharmacy staff assists other nurses. When it is her turn, the nurse receives the medication and returns to the floor. The dose is administered at 9:25 am, and the nurse spends the rest of the day trying to make up the lost 30 minutes.

This situation occurs thousands of times daily in hospitals around the United States. Neither the nurse nor the pharmacist is at fault here. Both are doing their best to provide excellent care to patients. Nevertheless, the nurse has just wasted 30 minutes on a problem that was preventable. The nurse and the pharmacist are working in a system in which problems like the missing medication are inevitable. The problems are built into the system.

Scenario 2: At 8:55 am, a hospital nurse goes to the medication room to get a 9 am dose and finds it in the patient's cassette. The pharmacist, who is located on the nursing unit, has already picked up the order, keyed it into the computer, and placed the medication in the patient's cassette. The nurse gives the medication to the patient at 8:57 am.

In scenario 2, the pharmacist is better located to serve the nurse. A system is in place that permits the pharmacist to quickly receive and fill new orders. The pharmacist can consult with nurses and physicians face-to-face if any questions arise. In addition, the pharmacist is able to develop better professional relationships with nurses and physicians. This can help reduce conflict and misunderstandings. The service in scenario 2 is better because the system is better. Chapter 9, Designing Pharmacy Services, discusses this topic in more detail.

Lean Management Processes

Lean is a set of philosophies and methods to add value to business processes by reducing waste and waits.[18] In healthcare, it attempts to fundamentally change thinking and transform behaviors, practices, and culture. It continually asks "what is the value provided in each step of the provision of health care. Anything that does not add value is changed or deleted.

"Lean is a cultural transformation that changes how an organization works; no one stays on the sidelines in the quest to discover how to improve the daily work. It requires new habits, new skills, and often a new attitude throughout the organization from senior management to front-line service providers. Lean is a journey, not a destination."[19]

In pharmacy, it has been used to improve medication compounding,[20] oncology,[21] clinical practice,[22] and medication use in nursing homes. [23] Kohlberg[24] describes the following common wastes in health care that Lean attempts to reduce:

- o   Defects in products or service delivery
- o   Poor use of inventory
- o   Avoidable waiting
- o   Unplanned breaks in processes
- o   Unnecessary motion and steps in processes
- o   Duplication of effort
- o   Overproduction of services and products
- o   Underutilized employees
- o   Poor communication
- o   Inefficient transportation processes

Quality Improvement

All well-run service organizations have some form of quality improvement system. Existing under a variety of names such as previously mentioned lean management and others like total quality management, continuous quality improvement, or six-sigma, they all have the following common features:

Improvement must be continuous. Proponents assume that the status quo is not sufficient to survive in the marketplace. Quality that is adequate now will not be enough in the near future. Quality can be enhanced by continually simplifying the service process, eliminating duplication, streamlining unnecessary actions, decreasing process time, and preventing errors.

Quality must be customer-centered (or patient-centered). All improvements must be recognized and valued by customers. Quality from the provider's viewpoint is only relevant in its relationship to the desires of customers.

Quality must be measured. There are two common sayings relating to this topic, "Only that which is measured is important;" and "Only that which is measured gets accomplished." These sayings mean that quality must be defined and measured. Only then will service providers make it a priority. And only then will providers be able to assess quality and improve it.

Solutions to problems should be multidisciplinary and interprofessional. Most quality deficiencies are not located within a single healthcare discipline or department. A medication error by a patient can be caused by actions by the pharmacist, technician, physician, insurer, or other person. Therefore, solutions to quality problems must cross organizational and professional lines.

Assume mistakes are part of the service system. Poorly designed systems set individuals up to make mistakes through overwork, inadequate training or tools to do the job, or a range of other causes. Quality indicators should be used to find and fix causes within the system that result in poor quality – not to punish people who make errors. People who make mistakes are not bad, only human. Therefore, the focus should be on identifying and fixing problems with the system.

A bad system will beat a good person every time.

— *W. Edwards Deming*

The steps involved in quality improvement (QI) are shown in Figure 4-2 These steps are PLAN, DO, STUDY, and ACT.

PLAN. Service providers plan a service improvement by consulting everyone involved in the process. In pharmacy, this might include technicians, nurses, managers, and physicians. These individuals discuss common and important problems in the system that hinder their ability to serve patients. The purpose is to solicit potential problems to target for QI interventions.

Once a problem is targeted, baseline quality indicators are identified and collected to compare with post-improvement measures. For instance, waiting times for filling new prescriptions might be chosen based upon patient and pharmacist complaints. The indicator, time from dropping off the prescription to picking it up, could be measured before and after any intervention. Averages and ranges for waiting time can be used by members of the QI team to develop new improvement strategies and adjust old ones.

Ideally, indicators should originate from data already being collected such as sales figures, customer complaint records, or employee surveys. The more difficult it is to collect quality indicators, the less likely they will be gathered. A basic understanding of statistical quality control techniques is also useful for everyone involved.

DO. After a problem is identified for improvement, an action plan is developed and put into place. A solution for reducing dispensing errors might consist of a new double check system prior to dispensing any prescription. Small scale implementation of QI strategies are typical. That way, problems with implementation that crop up are more easily resolved.

STUDY. As post-intervention data is collected, it is analyzed for success and unintentional consequences of the improvement. The purpose might be to see if the action plan was implemented as decided, to identify correctable flaws in planning and implementation, or to identify new problems within the system that needs an intervention.

Analysis is facilitated with QI tools like those seen in Figure 4-3. For instance, a Pareto chart might be used to total the number of dispensing errors in order of frequency according to their causes. A discovery that errors after the QI intervention are due more frequently to pharmacist interruptions might suggest a direction for future QI interventions.

ACT. Then, the entire process of monitoring and assessment starts over again. The purpose is to continually seek out problems within the system and resolve them. This reduces errors, waste, inefficiencies, and costs of serving the customer.

In any service system, feedback and accountability are essential. Most managers and employees know that "If it is not measured, it is not important." Therefore, when the quality of services is never systematically measured or assessed, there is little pressure to improve. QI makes assessment and improvement part of everyday practice.

SUMMARY

Good pharmacy services do not just happen. They require much effort on the part of leaders, managers, and pharmacists. Leaders set forth a vision of excellent services. Managers make certain that vision is followed through actions such as recruitment, training, and internal marketing. Pharmacists provide good services day in and day out by working hard, paying attention to detail, and staying alert for ways to meet the needs of patients.

Reference List

(1) Berry LL, Bendapudi N. Health Care: A Fertile Field for Service Research. Journal of Service Research 2007;10(2):111-122.

(2) Bates DW. Preventing medication errors: a summary. Am J Health Syst Pharm 2007;64(14 Suppl 9):S3-S9.

(3) Craig S, Crane VS, Hayman JN, Hoffman R, Hatwig CA. Developing a service excellence system for ambulatory care pharmacy services. Am J Health Syst Pharm 2001;58(17):1597-1606.

(4) Kennedy DM, Caselli RJ, Berry LL. A roadmap for improving healthcare service quality. J Healthc Manag 2011;56(6):385-400.

(5) Zeithaml VA, MJ. B. Services Marketing. 1st ed. New York: McGraw-Hill Companies Inc.; 1996.

(6) Zeithaml VA, Parasuraman A, Berry LL. Problems and Strategies in Services Marketing. Journal of Marketing 1985;49(Spring):33-46.

(7) Berry LL, Seiders K, Wilder SS. Innovations in access to care: a patient-centered approach. Ann Intern Med 2003;139(7):568-574.

(8) Jacobs S, Ashcroft D, Hassell K. Culture in community pharmacy organisations: what can we glean from the literature? J Health Organ Manag 2011;25(4):420-454.

(9) Clark BE, Mount JK. Pharmacy Service Orientation: a measure of organizational culture in pharmacy practice sites. Res Social Adm Pharm 2006;2(1):110-128.

(10) Michel R, Nicholas JA. Management commitment to service quality and service recovery performance. Intl J of Pharm & Health Mrkt 2010;4(1):84-103.

(11) White L, Klinner C. Service quality in community pharmacy: an exploration of determinants. Res Social Adm Pharm 2012;8(2):122-132.

(12) Ton Z. Why "good jobs" are good for retailers. Harv Bus Rev 2012;90(1-2):124-31, 154.

(13) Berry LL. On great service: A framework for action. Journal of Marketing 1998;62(2):123-125.

(14) Heskett JL, Jones TO, Loveman GW, Sasser WE, Schlesinger LA. Putting The Service-Profit Chain To Work. Harvard Business Review 1994;72(2):164-174.

(15) Schlesinger LA, Heskett JL. The service-driven service company. Harv Bus Rev 1991;69(5):71-81.

(16) Javier R, Brian M. Towards the measurement of internal service quality. Int J of Service Industry Mgmt 1995;6(3):64-83.

(17) Cost of Pharmacist Turnover. ASHP Member Center on Staffing HR&PW, editor. 2009. American Society of Health System Pharmacists.

(18) Lawal AK, Rotter T, Kinsman L et al. Lean management in health care: definition, concepts, methodology and effects reported (systematic review protocol). Syst Rev 2014;3:103.

(19) Toussaint JS, Berry LL. The promise of Lean in health care. Mayo Clin Proc 2013;88(1):74-82.

(20) Tilson V, Dobson G, Haas CE, Tilson D. Mathematical modeling to reduce waste of compounded sterile products in hospital pharmacies. Hosp Pharm 2014;49(7):616-627.

(21) Sullivan P, Soefje S, Reinhart D, McGeary C, Cabie ED. Using lean methodology to improve productivity in a hospital oncology pharmacy. Am J Health Syst Pharm 2014;71(17):1491-1498.

(22) Green CF, Crawford V, Bresnen G, Rowe PH. A waste walk through clinical pharmacy: how do the 'seven wastes' of Lean techniques apply to the practice of clinical pharmacists. Int J Pharm Pract 2014.

(23) Baril C, Gascon V, Brouillette C. Impact of technological innovation on a nursing home performance and on the medication-use process safety. J Med Syst 2014;38(3):22.

(24) Beata K, Jens JD, Brehmer PO. Measuring lean initiatives in health care services: issues and findings. Int J Productivity & Perf Mgmt 2006;56(1):7-24.

Chapter Questions

1. From your experiences, what do you think is the greatest cause for poor pharmacist service?

2. Discuss the role of pharmacist appearance in patient perceptions of service.

3. Relate the concept of the four I's of intangibility, inconsistency, inventory,

and inseparability to the importance of selecting pharmacy personnel.

4. Why might a pharmacy benefit from practicing internal marketing with its employees?

5. What barriers to providing the best possible service do the pharmacists in your practice setting face? Compare your answer with issues discussed in this chapter.

Activities

1. Read the mission statement of your pharmacy. How does it emphasize service to customers? Do you receive messages consistent with this mission from your boss and the other managers with whom you interact?

2. Ask 20 people to describe an instance in which they received especially bad service from a business. Group the responses into common categories of your choosing (e.g., a promise not kept). Organize the responses into a bar chart that shows the primary cause of poor service.

CHAPTER **9**

DESIGNING PHARMACY SERVICES

Objectives

After studying this chapter, the reader should be able to

- ○ Compare and contrast the production line approach and the empowerment approach to designing and managing pharmacy services
- ○ Explain the concept of service scripts and their value in providing excellent pharmacy services
- ○ List the steps involved in service recovery
- ○ Describe tools for visualizing pharmacy services
- ○ Discuss the purpose and components of a service blueprint

Every system is perfectly designed to get the results it gets

— Donald Berwick

America's health care system is neither healthy, caring, nor a system.

— Walter Cronkite

The job of pharmacists is to work with customers to help them achieve their desired outcomes, which may consist of a combination of good service, low cost, and effective care for their health needs. If a pharmacy is well managed, customers may continue to return again and again. However, competent management may not be enough to win customer business and loyalty. Service design is increasingly important in personalizing care and conveying value and excellence to customers.

In many situations, pharmacists fail to provide excellent services due to problems with poor service design. Pharmacy employees are often hard workers who want to help patients, but their hands are tied by poorly designed systems and inflexible policies and procedures. The design and management of pharmacy organizations determine the quality of services provided. Pharmacies that are well designed and run can meet the needs of customers effectively and efficiently. Poorly designed and managed pharmacies waste resources and effort, cost more to operate, and are less effective in serving patients.

Chase and Hayes[1] categorized the quality of service organizations as follows:

Available for service. Organizations that fall into this category look at services as necessary evils. Services are not an important part of the business strategy and are considered only as an afterthought. Management provides minimal support for service operations. Service employees are considered an expense to the organization, not an asset. The primary message from management regarding services is "Don't screw up."

Journeyman. Organizations in this category realize that they must provide services in order to compete. However, service is provided more in response to competitors than in response to customer needs. In other words, the goal is to make services minimally competitive. Over time, these organizations begin to resemble their competitors. As in the previous category, employees are considered an expense to the organization, not an asset.

Distinctive competence. Organizations in this category have a customer focus and continually work to meet customer needs. Service is an integral part of organizational strategy, and resources are committed to providing excellent service. Employees are considered assets to the firm, because they are important in attracting and keeping customers. Customers recognize that the service is different from that of competitors.

World-class service delivery. Organizations in this category are considered not only excellent but innovative. Employees are treated as assets because they generate revenue and are a source of innovations. At the same time, employee performance standards are very demanding. World-class service companies set the standard for all others.

Most likely, there are pharmacy organizations in each of these categories, although few can survive for long in the first two categories. This chapter describes how pharmacy organizations can design and manage services in ways that help the organization stand out from competitors.

APPROACHES TO SERVICE DESIGN

Two broad approaches occur in the design and management of excellent service.[2] The production line approach attempts to standardize service performance, simplify tasks, and keep decision-making authority in the hands of management. In contrast, the empowerment approach encourages employees to take greater responsibility for their jobs and to exercise initiative in performing them. This approach attempts to motivate employees to act independently to give excellent, individualized service to each customer.

Production Line Approach

The *production line approach* is based on the philosophy that customers' needs can best be met with services that are efficient, low cost, and consistent. In production line organizations, management designs the service system, and employees provide the services exactly as designed. A top-down approach is used, and employees are required to act as cogs in a smoothly running service machine. Management's goals are to standardize service performance, simplify tasks, provide a clear division of labor, substitute equipment and systems for employees when possible, and minimize the need for employees to make independent decisions.[3, 4]

McDonald's is a well-known example of production line organization in the fast food business. The McDonald's strategy is to make every restaurant in the chain provide the same high-quality food and service. The service employees typically are low-wage, low-skilled workers who are trained to do exactly what they are taught in cooking the food and serving the customers. Each employee has a simple, clearly defined task that is to be done quickly and efficiently. When possible, technology is used to simplify the task and replace employees. Independent decisions by employees (e.g., offering to place blue cheese on a cheeseburger, giving a free meal to good customers) are discouraged.

Production line approaches can be found in high-prescription-volume pharmacies such as mail order and online pharmacies. Dispensing tasks are standardized and simplified as much as possible. The responsibilities of pharmacists and technicians are clearly divided, with technicians attempting to free up the pharmacists for more complex tasks. When possible, robots, automated telephone systems, Internet services, dispensing machines, computers, and other technology are substituted for employees. Staffing is kept to a minimum, so little time may be available for pharmacists to make professional decisions or provide individualized services to patients.

In production line pharmacies, efficiency is demanded of employees. Service is defined in terms of speed and accuracy of dispensing. The greater the efficiency, the lower is the personnel cost per prescription dispensed. An additional benefit of the production line approach is that tasks are simplified so that employees can be quickly trained and easily replaced if they quit. In pharmacy chains that use the production line approach, simplification and standardization permit employees to be moved from pharmacy to pharmacy, depending on the immediate need. Managers can use pharmacists and technicians as interchangeable parts of the service system.

Empowerment Approach

An alternative to a production line is the *empowerment approach*. The nature of services (i.e., intangibility, simultaneous consumption and production, heterogeneity, perishability) has caused many managers and scholars to argue that service workers should be given significant discretion in how they deal with customers.[2, 5, 6] They argue that the interactive nature of services requires that workers be permitted to make prompt and independent decisions to meet each customer's needs. If workers are given the authority and resources, they can identify and correct potential problems before they happen, correct service failures once they occur, and be responsive to the dynamics of service situations.

Empowerment is the term commonly used for giving employees increased authority and flexibility in how they do their jobs. Definitions of empowerment vary, but most agree that empowerment means employees are permitted to exercise some degree of discretion in the delivery of services.[7] Instead of limiting employee actions with strict policies and procedures for the correct way to serve customers, employees are given discretion in how to best serve customers.

Compared with the production line approach, empowered employees have greater responsibility in the provision of service. Empowered employees do not say, "It's not my job" when customer problems occur. They take charge of resolving problems and finding ways to prevent future difficulties.

The empowerment approach assumes that frontline service workers know more than management does about serving individual customers. Therefore, workers are freed from unnecessary rules and regulations that constrain their ability to act in the customer's best interest. One problem with rigid policies and procedures is that they can reduce employee risk taking, leading employees to use policies as an excuse for not helping customers. Most people have faced a service employee who says "It's against our policy" in response to some simple request. In that organization, it is probably easier and safer for the employee to tell a customer "no" rather than risk breaking a policy. Doing the right thing for a customer is often riskier than blindly adhering to inflexible rules.

Excellent service organizations empower their employees to do what is necessary to serve the customer, without substantial constraints. At one department store renowned for its service, the employee handbook gives the following directions for dealing with customers: "Rule 1: Use your good judgment in all situations. There are no additional rules." This is a strong statement by management that employees are empowered to decide how to best serve customers, rather than consult management about what is appropriate.

Benefits of Empowerment

Table 9-1 lists benefits of the empowerment approach.[7] One of the main benefits is that employees can provide individualized services in response to the unique needs of customers. In each service situation, there are "moments of truth" in which a customer can be gained or lost. The empowerment approach permits employees to respond quickly to opportunities to provide excellent service and solve problems resulting from poor service. Decisions do not need to be made through the manager.

It is hard for managers to encourage exceptional services through policies and procedures, because policies and procedures cannot address all service situations. Instead, exceptional services are accomplished because frontline employees want to serve their customers and are able to do so. The following conditions are often associated with exceptional services.[8]

- *Adaptability of employees.* Adaptability refers to the flexibility of employees in responding to customer needs and requests. Customers appreciate it when service providers expend extra effort to adapt to special needs or requests. This differs from situations in which providers quote rules that limit their ability to provide anything beyond the norm. Sometimes, being adaptable even means breaking the rules. For example, it may be necessary for a pharmacist to dispense an emergency drug without all of the necessary documentation. It may break the rules, but in some situations it can be the most appropriate course of action.

- *Spontaneity of employee actions.* Customers often appreciate unprompted and unsolicited employee actions, such as an offer to deliver a medication to a patient's home or an offer to help choose a nonprescription cold medication. Customers remember spontaneous actions by employees that result in special attention or some other bonus.

- *An employee's ability to cope.* Employees who can handle difficult situations without losing their composure (i.e., demonstrate grace under pressure) are associated with exceptional services. For example, pharmacists reveal poor coping skills by snapping at co-workers or patients when the workload gets heavy. Pharmacists with good coping skills maintain their composure no matter how heavy the workload.

o *Recovery.* Recovery refers to an employee's response to a failure in service delivery. A pharmacist's response after a dispensing error, running out of a drug, or not meeting a promise is one of the most critical factors in determining whether a customer remains loyal to a service provider.[9-11] When a pharmacist or pharmacy makes a mistake, the response can help recover any respect, confidence, or faith that has been lost.

TABLE 9-1 Benefits and Costs of the Empowerment Approach

Benefits	Costs
Better capacity to respond to the unique needs of customers	Slower service
More individualized service	Potentially higher labor costs
Better ability to quickly resolve problems	Employees cannot be easily interchanged
Greater sense of employee ownership about their jobs	Less easy to replace employees with part-timers
Greater employee acceptance of responsibility for service and outcomes	Technology is less able to replace empowered employees, because their output is less standardized (for technology to be used, standardization of tasks is necessary)
Lower turnover, absenteeism, presence of trade unions	
More employee warmth and enthusiasm in customer interactions	Greater need for flexible and competent leadership
Positive customer word of mouth recommendations and loyalty	Employers have to be willing to accept that empowered employees will sometimes make bad decisions

Source: Reference [7]

Empowerment can make employees feel better about their jobs.[7] Empowerment by management demonstrates respect for employees. It says that management trusts the capabilities of employees enough to share responsibility with them and treat them as valued adults. Empowerment also increases feelings of ownership; this results in better feelings about the job itself. Think about how people differ in their treatment of a house they rent and one they own. With ownership, people take greater pride in their home and spend more time on maintenance and repair. The same is true about job ownership. Employees who feel ownership of a job take greater interest in what they do and how well it is done. Ownership enhances employee feelings about the job because it increases the perception that the employee's work has meaning. Employees who feel good about their jobs show greater warmth and enthusiasm when they interact with customers.

Costs of Empowerment

Table 9-1 also lists costs of the empowerment approach. Empowerment requires more leadership from management. Rather than directing employees to accomplish tasks, managers need to inspire employees to take responsibility for the job. This can be difficult for managers who are used to working in a production line system. It requires them to be teachers, coaches, and team leaders.

Managers also need to change employee attitudes about work. Many employees have never had to accept responsibility for their work. Employees need to realize that they will be held accountable for more than just showing up. They need to understand that their performance and rewards will be assessed against measures of group output. For example, pharmacist and technician performance may be evaluated with measures such as pharmacy profitability, number of repeat customers, and sales volume.

Employees need sufficient information about their jobs if they are to share responsibility with management.[2, 7] They need information that will help them appreciate where their job fits within the overall context of the organization, because many service decisions depend on understanding the consequences of different courses of action. For example, a pharmacist who does not charge a patient for a prescription needs to understand the financial impact that will have on the organization.

Another cost of the empowerment approach is that it is often less efficient and can result in service that is slower and more expensive. With production line organizations, labor costs per unit of output tend to be lower.

Finally, empowered employees can make bad decisions. It is possible to go too far in pleasing customers. A pharmacist may decide to solve a conflict by offering to give the customer a $50 prescription at no charge. With loyal customers, it may be good business sense to generate goodwill that results in future revenue. But the $50 can be a significant portion of the day's profit for the pharmacy and may never result in any customer goodwill.

WHICH APPROACH IS BETTER?

Most pharmacies use a combination of the empowerment and production line approaches to provide service. Even the most empowered employees need structure in their jobs. On the other hand, it is impossible to control every aspect of employee behavior in production line pharmacies. Still, many pharmacies lean toward one approach or another when serving customers.

So, which approach is better? The answer depends on several factors:[7]

o   Basic business strategy. If a pharmacy's business strategy is to provide low-cost, high-volume services, then a production line approach is preferred. If the business strategy is based on personalized, customized services, then an empowerment approach is better.

o   Nature of the transaction. If most transactions between pharmacists and patients are single, discrete transactions, then a production line approach is better. If numerous transactions over a long time period lead to a pharmacist–patient therapeutic relationship, then an empowerment approach is preferred.

o   Needs of the patients. Patients who have complex medical needs can benefit from services founded on an empowerment approach. If drug-related problems are routine and simple, a production line approach may be sufficient.

o   Type of employees and managers. Each of these approaches works best with certain types of managers and employees. The production line approach works better for managers who prefer to monitor and control employees. Such managers may not feel comfortable sharing responsibility with employees. The production line approach also works when employees do not want to be empowered. Some pharmacy employees are more comfortable working in production line jobs that consist of routine tasks, easy-to-solve problems, and no-risk situations. The empowerment approach demands managers who are willing and able to help employees accept greater responsibility. This requires excellent leadership and coaching skills. In addition, the empowerment approach requires employees who want to take responsibility for their jobs and are bored and unchallenged with repetitive, routine tasks.

The answer to which approach is better comes down to a tradeoff between management control over the service process and employee involvement in services.[7] If management believes that greater control over the process will result in better customer value, then a production line approach may be preferable. On the other hand, if greater employee involvement in services is desired, then an empowerment approach should be used.

INDUSTRIALIZED INTIMACY

Industrialized intimacy has been proposed as an alternative service design to the two extremes of production-line and empowerment approaches.[12] Industrialized intimacy seeks to blend technology with empowered workers to achieve a high level of contact, communication, and coordination with customers. Collecting data on customers and making it available at a touch to service workers can build a high level of customer intimacy. With technology, pharmacists can have easy access to information about patient therapy, service preferences, insurance coverage, and best practices. In addition to being effective in meeting needs, it can be highly efficient.

Pharmacies that can integrate information and service technology into delivery processes create personalized, high-quality service with the efficiency of a production line approach. Increasingly, this model of service design is becoming a standard of practice.

For example, a retired school teacher might fill a prescription at Walgreens. From information collected and maintained by Walgreens, the pharmacist can monitor the retiree's drug use and medical history over time. The retiree has her prescription sent electronically to Walgreens which is filled and ready for dispensing upon arrival. The teacher is sent automatic reminders to refill her prescriptions, and pharmacists at Walgreens monitor her medication profile for harmful drug interactions and other drug related problems. Service is offered 24/7 via Internet, mobile devices, 24-hour pharmacies, and call centers. If needed, specialty pharmacy and medication therapy management services are available for complex medical needs.

Service design using industrialized intimacy follows seven principles:[12]

1. Know your customer. Detailed knowledge of each pharmacy customer allows pharmacists and other employees personalize services with efficiency and effectiveness. A call to the pharmacy might go like this: "Thank you for calling Forest Hill Pharmacy. Can I have your name? It's good to hear from you again Mr. Smith. How can I help you today? Yes, I can refill your lovastatin prescription early so you can go on vacation. I noticed that your thiazide prescription should run out in the next week. Have you been taking it consistently? Do you want me

to refill that prescription too? OK. We'll make certain that the prescriptions will be filled in electronic reminder bottles as usual. Is there anything else I can do for you? Have a good day! Good Bye."

2. Strive for once-and-done servicing. This means eliminating or minimizing the number of handoffs required to complete a transaction. In pharmacy, it might mean having collaborative practice agreements with physicians to automatically take care of common problems without continually having to contact them.

3. Promote value-enhancing self-servicing. This means using self-service technology when possible to perform tasks. It gives customers greater control and can reduce aggravation associated with waiting.

4. Provide one-stop shopping. Pharmacies have mastered this strategy by identifying customer shopping needs and meeting those needs within a single store or online shopping experience.

5. Let customers design the product or service. This is a variation on patient-centered care where providers provide patients with service options and letting them choose. Depending on patient engagement, their participation can be extensive or minimal.

6. Engineer competency into service delivery. This requires service design that employ continuous quality improvement and Lean design principles. These issues are discussed later in the chapter.

7. Build long-term customer relationships. If the previous six principles are followed, customers will want to continue to return to the pharmacy. They will receive exceptional value for their health care dollar.

SERVICE EXPERIENCE

When designing pharmacy services, it is important to have an intimate understanding of the customers' service experience. The *service experience* describes the steps customers that go through when interacting with a business.[26] For pharmacies, the experience might be online, in a store, over the phone, in a hospital, or any combination of interactions of the provision of service. The service experience is often referred to as the "customer journey", and journeys are described with customer journey maps.[27]

Customer journeys are made up of multiple *touch-points*; the points of contact between a service provider and customers.[28] A pharmacy service journey might include series of touch-points including customer experiences with the pharmacy parking lot, the pharmacy building itself, signage, website, phone calls, printed bag, self-service machines, and contact with front-line employees like clerks, technicians, and pharmacists. Each time a customer interacts with a touch-point, they have a service-encounter. The more touchpoints, the more complex is the service experience (or service journey).

Thinking about pharmacy services in terms of journeys can help pharmacists take a more holistic approach to the customer experience. Services are viewed as an overall experience instead of discrete events. Mapping the journey is a way of understanding that experience and identifying gaps in the customer journey.

There is no single way of mapping the customer journey but most contain the following steps:

1. Identify all of the people who will be involved in the service experience in some way. This might include patients, physicians, techs, pharmacists, and billing people.

2. From the patient's viewpoint, list all of the steps that need to be completed to receive the service. These steps might include pre-purchase steps (identifying the need for a service), purchase steps (going to the pharmacy), and post-purchase steps (taking the medication as directed). Often, this step is facilitated by developing *customer personas*--archetypes of targeted customers. Personas represent who customers are, what they want, their goals, how they think, how they shop, and why they purchase.

3. List all of the points of contact between the patient and specific employees. Also list touch-points with technology (self-service) and inanimate objects (parking lot).

4. List the services that are provided in the pharmacy and a visible to the patient.

5. List all of the support services provided to the frontline employees and the backstage people providing them. This might include housekeeping, information support, and financial offices.

6. Now map the elements on the outline using a formal structure like flow charts, diagrams, or service blueprints (described later in this chapter).

7. Identify *moments of truth* from the map. These are key touch-points which have exceptional impact on the service experience (e.g., face-to-face interactions with the pharmacist).

PLANNING FOR SERVICE PERFORMANCE

"The best way to predict the future is to design it."

– Buckminster Fuller

The quality of pharmacy services can be enhanced through better planning and design. Common strategies used in the design of services are presented here.

Service Scripts

Service scripts are used by businesses to help employees learn how to perform service duties and to standardize certain aspects of performance. A service script describes service performance in a written list of actions.[13] The following example is a service script for handling a penicillin-allergic patient who presents a prescription for a cephalosporin.

1. A penicillin-allergic patient presents a cephalosporin prescription.

2. The pharmacist questions the patient about details of the allergy to ascertain whether the patient actually has an allergy and the severity of the allergic reaction.

3. The pharmacist calls the physician to discuss the risks of dispensing the drug, possible alternatives for the patient, and directions for the patient.

4. The pharmacist initiates the agreed-upon action plan and documents the plan on the prescription.

The service script establishes the expected actions and responsibilities of the parties involved in performing the service. This example defines the problem (i.e., a penicillin-allergic patient presenting a prescription for a drug that may cause an allergic reaction), lists steps to be taken to solve the problem, and assigns responsibility for each step. There is little doubt about what is expected of the pharmacist.

The service script standardizes how employees handle problems. Standardization can reduce confusion for both the service provider and the customer. Imagine what would happen if a pharmacist did not document physician consultation about a prescription. A co-worker might duplicate a previous consultation by calling a physician about a problem that had already been solved. This would waste both the physician's and the pharmacist's time and cause the physician to wonder about the pharmacist's competence.

Service scripts should reflect the best known methods for handling service situations. Scripts should be developed by experienced service employees who can share their expertise. Input should also be solicited from employees who might be expected to follow the scripts. The scripts themselves should be comprehensive enough to help guide the actions of employees without constraining their ability to take care of customers.

Service scripts can be used in both production line and empowerment organizations. The difference lies in how they are used. In production line organizations, service scripts can be used as strict guidelines for employee behavior when dealing with customers. Here, scripts are followed without change or judgment. In empowerment organizations, scripts are used as a tool for training employees in unfamiliar tasks. They are used to suggest behavior, not as instructions to be followed exactly as written. As employees gain experience with the scripted task, they should be encouraged to move beyond it—to inject their own personality and experience into the service performance. This leads the employee to interpret and redefine the script, just as an actor does with the script of a play.

Many pharmacy schools use scripts in teaching their students. One example is the Indian Health Service guidelines for counseling patients. These guidelines require asking patients three questions:

1. What did the doctor tell you the medicine is for?
2. How did the doctor tell you to take the medicine?
3. What did the doctor tell you to expect?

This simple script helps new pharmacists learn how to acquire basic information from patients that can be used in therapeutic problem solving. With experience, pharmacists can develop their own interpretation of the script, based on their own practice setting and experience.

Service scripts can relate to almost any situation, including clinical problems and basic work activities. New pharmacists might benefit from scripts dealing with the following: a dispensing error, a situation that requires a physician to change a prescribed therapy, a non-formulary prescription, a prior authorization, a nursing administration error, a patient complaint about the price of a prescription, a drug incompatibility, a physician prescribing error, a drug allergy or drug interaction, a service mistake (e.g., overcharge), negotiation with co-workers, a difficult counseling situation, a patient with renal or hepatic insufficiency, or a hostile customer.

Planning for Service Recovery

Many organizations have scripts for dealing with failures in service. All of us have experienced bad service. We may have had to wait too long for service or received merchandise we did not order. Bad service is a fact of life in business.

Providing bad service can hurt a firm's image. People are more likely to remember bad service than good service. Bad service colors customer impressions of a firm, leads to negative comments about the experience, and drives customers to competitors.[14]

Failures can occur at numerous points in the service delivery process. Events within a service experience that determine the customer's overall evaluation of the service are called *critical incidents*. Critical incidents that are perceived as negative by the customer are called service failures. Service failures in pharmacy include incorrect charges for merchandise, unusually slow service, out-of-stock drugs, rude and uncooperative employees, and dispensing errors.

Customers respond to service failures in a number of ways. One way is to complain. Customers who complain are those who care enough to let an organization know that they are dissatisfied with some aspect of service. Complainers can actually be an organization's best friends, because they pinpoint problems in the service system that could lead to the loss of customers. Only a small fraction of customers complain, however.

Dissatisfied customers who do not complain show their displeasure with service failures in other ways. One way is to quit doing business with the company. These customers may make a conscious decision to never patronize a business again, or gradually move their business to competitors over time. In worst-case scenarios, they retaliate and try to hurt the business in some way. They may go out of their way to complain to others about the poor service (e.g., setting up a Web site to share service "horror stories" about a company), take legal action, or even resort to vandalism against the business.

Service Recovery

The costs of negative service can be significant, and many organizations develop ways to address the problem of service failure. One important strategy is to design systems that minimize the number of service failures. Since it is impossible to prevent all bad experiences, businesses often have plans to minimize the impact of service failure.

Service recovery refers to all actions taken by personnel in a firm in response to a service failure. For example, if a customer notices that you have overcharged him for a drug by $10, just correcting the charge may not be enough to satisfy him. Although your action may fix the problem, it won't necessarily win the customer back. The customer may assume that if you are sloppy with charges, you also may be sloppy in filling prescriptions. As a result, he probably will be wary of you and conduct future business elsewhere.

When a service failure does occur, most service recovery programs use the following steps to help the customer feel good about doing business in the future:[15]

1. Offer an apology. When making an apology, first acknowledge that an error has been made and then acknowledge any inconvenience or concern it has caused. This lets the patient know that you recognize his or her situation and are concerned. Then take responsibility for remedying the situation. No matter who made the error or why it was made, you must convey concern for the customer and willingness to resolve the problem. Customers usually are not interested in reasons for the problem. What most people want to hear is, simply, "I'm truly sorry for the error."

2. Offer a remedy. It is important to follow up an apology with a solution that tells the customer you are concerned about his or her well-being and future patronage. Listen to the customer's assessment of the problem, and find a solution that will address every concern the customer expresses. For example, if the customer seems to be concerned about future mischarges, explain how similar mistakes will be prevented in the future.

3. Fix the problem immediately. Drop everything, and make solving this problem a priority. Doing so reinforces your dedication to resolving the problem and preserving the patient relationship. Acting assertively yet compassionately is crucial.

4. Offer some form of compensation for the patient's inconvenience. This step is not always necessary. For small failures, an apology may be enough. However, some compensation, such as forgoing a copayment or filling the prescription at no charge, can let the customer know that (1) you consider the mistake unacceptable, (2) it won't happen again, and (3) you care about keeping his or her business. Companies that have compensation as a part of their normal method of handling errors will either have to prevent errors from occurring or lose business through giveaways.

The surprising result of competent and sincere service recovery is that customers often feel better about the experience than if no service failure had occurred.[15] This is because failures give the service provider an opportunity to provide exceptional service. If the service provider performs well, the customer will recall the entire event in a positive light.

It is important to note that service recovery works only when service failures are rare. If a company has frequent failures in core services, customers will stop doing business with it, no matter what compensation is offered.

MARKETING IN ACTION

Why Not Slow Meds?

Why is it so important for patients to get their medications so fast? Why do pharmacies all have drive-thru windows and express counters? Doesn't this discourage interactions between pharmacists and patients?

Some design experts think so.[16, 17] They wonder why visits to pharmacies mirror a visit to McDonalds to pick up a double cheeseburger.

Design experts argue that the push for fast medications misses an opportunity for the health care system.[16, 17] Despite the fact that the average patient interacts with his or her pharmacist 12 to 15 times a year, few have a relationship with their pharmacist. And although pharmacists are the most accessible professionals, few patients turn to their pharmacist for help with their medication needs.

Fast meds are the antithesis of the old days of neighborhood pharmacies and apothecaries, which were warm and inviting places for patients to chat and consult with their personal pharmacist. In their attempt to speed up the delivery of medications, community pharmacists have lost the special something they used to have to help people.[17]

One design expert says that pharmacists can learn a lot from traditional Chinese medicine shops. When visiting a shop in Taiwan, the expert found the containers of exotic herbs and powdered animal parts to be a little scary, but most interesting was the 45-minute conversation he had with the "pharmacist." The pharmacist took the time to talk, listen, and explain about Chinese medicine. His encounter was more extensive and informative than any conversation ever received by a pharmacist in the United States.

Although some will dismiss the idea behind Chinese medicine or argue that spending 45 minutes with patients is impossible, U.S. pharmacists and pharmacies can do more to encourage conversation. And some now are.

Select Walgreens pharmacies have been redesigned to appear more like an Apple Genius Bar, than a traditional pharmacy. Pharmacists are stationed at an "Ask Your Pharmacist" booth to guide patients to the dispensing area, private consultation room, or the nursing care clinic. The result is better communications with pharmacists.

Walgreens new design is the exception to what most customers see because pharmacies are paid for pushing pills, not helping patients take those pills correctly. That has lead to a system of pharmacy practice that encourages pharmacists to dispense more and more medications while doing little to deal with patient confusion and non-adherence.

Designers have suggestions for developing next-generation pharmacies.[16, 17] One opportunity occurs during the critical time after a new diagnosis when patients are hurting both physically and emotionally. Pharmacists can help patients to adapt to a new life with illness when patients are most likely to be actively seeking information and guidance. The first six months after diagnosis provides the best opportunity for pharmacists to build a lasting relationship with customers.

Another opportunity lies in targeting the growing number of baby boomers seeking help with medication therapy management. Pharmacists can act as health centers for health promotion and disease management -- offering an individualized mix of healthcare services and merchandise.

Source: References [16, 17]

VISUALIZING PHARMACIST SERVICES

Complex systems pharmacist services are easier to understand and evaluate when they are put into a visual form such as with a flowchart or diagram.[18, 19] The three most common forms of visualization processes in pharmacy are flowcharts, supply chain diagrams, and service blueprints.

Flowcharts

Flowcharts are used to visually describe processes in businesses, data processing, and health care. These process charts typically include geometric symbols (e.g., diamond, oval) that represent various steps in a process (e.g., handoffs, inspection). They are so common that most basic productivity software, like word processing programs, have functions to develop flowcharts. Flowcharting is common in medication use design.[20-22] An example is shown in Figure 9.1.

Figure 9.1 Example of a Flowchart of the dispensing process

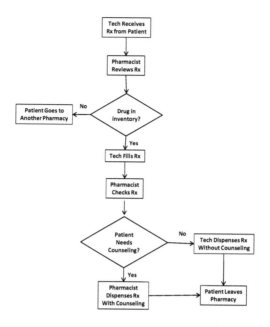

Supply Chain Diagrams

Supply chain diagrams, illustrated in Figure 9.2, show relationships between elements of a process.

Figure 9-2 Example of a Supply Chain Diagram

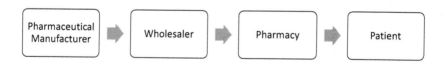

Service Blueprints

The workflow in service organizations can have a tremendous impact on the quality and efficiency of services. Often, flowcharts called service blueprints are used to map the steps of service delivery.

Service blueprints permit service providers to better see and understand service processes. A service blueprint depicts the process of service delivery and the roles of customers, service providers, and supporting services. It breaks down the service into components and arranges them according to their purpose. An example of a service blueprint is shown in Figure 9-3.

Service blueprints are based on process design theory from industrial engineering and operations management.[23, 24] A key feature unique to service blueprinting is the inclusion of customers and their view of the process. The premise of service blueprints is that if customers contribute to the service process, they should be recognized explicitly in its design and management. This means that the customer's "job" must be clearly defined.

The primary benefit of service blueprints is that they force a careful analysis of each step in the service process and help communicate that information to people such as the frontline employees who help determine its success.

Components of a Service Blueprint

There are no concrete rules for designing service blueprints, so the process can be very flexible. However, service blueprints have some key components:[25] customer actions, "onstage" contact employee actions, "backstage" contact employee actions, and support processes, as shown in Figure 9-3.

Customer actions are performed by the customer, who can be any recipient of service (e.g., physician, nurse, patient), depending on the process. Customer actions in pharmacy include face-to-face consultation with pharmacists and telephone calls for prescription refills.

Customer actions are matched by onstage and backstage employee actions. Onstage employee actions are visible to the customer. The patient can see the pharmacist or technician taking the prescription and the pharmacist providing counseling. Anything done for the patient that is not visible is a backstage employee action. Backstage actions include professional decisions made by pharmacists, such as checking the patient profile for drug allergies, interactions, and duplicate medications or consulting with the physician about therapy.

Support processes are those that support contact employees in the delivery of services. For pharmacists, these might include computer support services, billing, development of patient education inserts, and inventory control.

The service blueprint components are separated by three horizontal lines: the line of interaction, the line of visibility, and the line of internal interaction. The line of interaction is where customers and providers interact. Service encounters occur wherever a vertical line crosses the line of interaction. The line of visibility separates onstage contact employee actions and backstage employee actions. Actions below this line are invisible to the customer. This line is critical, because patients' image of a pharmacist is determined to a great extent by what they see the pharmacist do. If the primary patient view is of the pharmacist counting and pouring, then the image of pharmacists will be consistent with that view. The line of internal interaction separates frontline employees from supporting individuals. Any line that crosses this line indicates a process that supports the frontline employee.

Figure 9-3 Service Blueprint of a Smoking Cessation Program

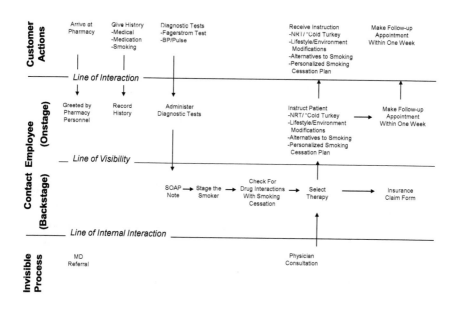

NRT = nicotine replacement therapy; SOAP = subjective and objective findings, assessment, and plan. "Claim Form" refers to the National Community Pharmacists Association pharmacist claim form and Centers for Medicare and Medicaid Services forms.

Building a Blueprint

Before a blueprint can be designed, a service process must be selected. An entire service process (e.g., dispensing) can be mapped, or the focus can be on a specific component of the process (e.g., patient counseling). An overview of the entire service process is called a concept blueprint.26 Concept blueprints demonstrate how each job or department functions in relation to the process as a whole. Detailed blueprints can be used to clarify components identified in the concept blueprint.

Insight and understanding are gained through the development of a service blueprint. Building a blueprint requires those involved to explicitly evaluate each step in the service process. This analysis encourages communication between designers, with several possible benefits. It can help clarify the service steps and identify obstacles that were not initially apparent. It can also help delineate the roles and responsibilities of each participant in the service process, even those who are not traditionally thought of as participants (e.g., customers, supporting services). Finally, it can foster a shared vision among all involved.

Since pharmacy blueprints encompass customers, pharmacists, technicians, managers, and supporting staff, all of these people should have input in blueprint development. Most critical, however, is understanding how customers view a service. A customer focus permits designers to highlight processes that accentuate customer value.

There are five steps to building a service blueprint:[25]

1.   Identify the process to be blueprinted. Service blueprints should be designed with a specific purpose in mind. A concept blueprint might be used for understanding an overall process. To address specific problem areas of a service, a detailed blueprint might be more appropriate.

2.   Map the process from the customer's point of view. Each action and choice of the customer is charted—not only those steps involved in purchasing a service but also those involved in consuming and evaluating it. This helps focus on the processes that affect customer perceptions.

3.   Map contact employee actions. Mapping both onstage and backstage employee actions provides an opportunity for service employees and managers to communicate. Care must be taken to ensure that each term in the service blueprint has the same meaning for everyone, especially if there is opportunity for different interpretations. For example, it may be wise to define "patient counseling" in any blueprint. A line of interaction and a line of visibility should be drawn separating customer and employee actions and onstage and backstage employee actions, respectively.

4. Map internal support activities. The line of internal interaction should be drawn and linkages between contact and support employees should be diagrammed.

5. Add evidence of service at each customer action step. The physical evidence of service can be mapped to illustrate what the customer sees and experiences during each contact with the pharmacy.

A service blueprint helps pharmacy managers identify potential problem areas in the service process. For example, a blueprint of a smoking cessation program is shown in Figure 9-3. It allows the pharmacist to review key elements of the program experience for potential obstacles. The pharmacist may discover that problems occur with data collection or interactions with the physician. The blueprint allows the pharmacist to see each step in the process, probe for difficulties, and identify problem areas.

A blueprint also facilitates analysis of cost–benefit tradeoffs in designing services. For example, the level of pharmacist–customer contact is critical. A pharmacy that stresses efficiency in services may find it efficient to limit patient–pharmacist interactions, because pharmacists can complete more work when they are not interrupted by telephone calls and patient questions. On the other hand, a customer-driven pharmacy may find that the greater the contact, the greater is the opportunity to develop a patient relationship and demonstrate the value of pharmacist services. The blueprint provides a template for quantifying the value of patient contact, as measured by repeat customers, patient satisfaction, and out-comes of drug therapy.

A blueprint also helps employees visualize the entire service process. It enables each employee to better understand his or her role in the process, how that role affects others in the process, and exactly what is to be achieved by everyone on the team. Including employees in the blueprinting process can increase their buy-in to operational changes or new service development by giving them the opportunity to provide feedback in the planning stages instead of during implementation.

Pharmacy services must be designed with customer value and satisfaction in mind. Each design step should be assessed for its contribution to the customer's perception of value, as well as its contribution to positive patient outcomes. Steps that do not provide value should be reconsidered or omitted.

SUMMARY

Service design can make the difference between poor and excellent pharmacy services. The production line and empowerment approaches to the provision of services can both be useful frameworks. The choice of approach depends on the basic business strategy, the nature of the pharmacy transaction, the needs of patients, and the people employed by the pharmacy.

No matter which approach is chosen, pharmacists can benefit from techniques developed in other service industries. Service scripts can be developed to establish the expected actions and responsibilities of service employees. Service blueprints can be used to map the steps involved in service delivery. Service audits provide systematic, critical reviews of the role and performance of marketing within organizations.

Reference List

(1) Chase RB, Hayes RH. Beefing up operations in service firms. Sloan Manage Rev 1991;33(1):15-26.

(2) Bowen DE, Lawler EE, III. The empowerment of service workers: what, why, how, and when. Sloan Manage Rev 1992;33(3):31-39.

(3) Levitt T. Industrialization of Servce. Harv Bus Rev 1976;(Sept.-Oct.):63-74.

(4) Levitt T. Production line approach to service. Harv Bus Rev 1972;(Sept.-Oct.):41-52.

(5) Berry LL, Seiders K, Wilder SS. Innovations in access to care: a patient-centered approach. Ann Intern Med 2003;139(7):568-574.

(6) Schlesinger LA, Heskett JL. The service-driven service company. Harv Bus Rev 1991;69(5):71-81.

(7) Bowen DE, Lawler EE. Empowering Service Employees. Sloan Management Review 1995;36(4):73-84.

(8) Zeithaml VA, MJ. B. Services Marketing. 1st ed. New York: McGraw-Hill Companies Inc.; 1996.

(9) Michel R, Nicholas JA. Management commitment to service quality and service recovery performance. Intl J of Pharm & Health Mrkt 2010;4(1):84-103.

(10) Smith AK, Bolton RN, Wagner J. A model of customer satisfaction with service encounters involving failure and recovery. Journal of Marketing Research 1999;36(3):356-372.

(11) Hart CW, Heskett JL, Sasser WE, Jr. The profitable art of service recovery. Harv Bus Rev 1990;68(4):148-156.

(12) Kolesar P, Van Rysin G, Cutler W. Creating customer value through industrialized intimacy. Strategy and Business 1998;July 1(12).

(13) Holdford D. Service scripts: a tool for teaching pharmacy students how to handle common practice situations. Am J Pharm Educ 2006;70(1):2.

(14) Zeithaml VA, Berry LL, Parasuraman A. The behavioral consequences of service quality. Journal of Marketing 1996;60(2):31-46.

(15) Tax SS, Brown SW. Recovering and learning from service failure. Sloan Management Review 1998;40(1):75-88.

(16) Hirsch J. A Wellness Disaster: Pharmacies Modeled On Fast Food Joints. FastCompany . 8-27-2012.

(17) Formosa D. One Fix For Health Care: Dissolving The Barrier Between Patients And Pharmacists. Fast Company . 7-10-2012.

(18) Emmett D, Paul DP, Chandra A, Barrett H. Pharmacy layout: What are consumers' perceptions? J Hosp Mark Public Relations 2006;17(1):67-77.

(19) McDowell AL, Huang YL. Selecting a pharmacy layout design using a weighted scoring system. Am J Health Syst Pharm 2012;69(9):796-804.

(20) Goudswaard AN, Stolk RP, de Valk HW, Rutten GE. Improving glycaemic control in patients with Type 2 diabetes mellitus without insulin therapy. Diabet Med 2003;20(7):540-544.

(21) Parry MF, Stewart J, WRIGHT P, McLeod GX. Collaborative management of HIV infection in the community: an effort to improve the quality of HIV care. AIDS Care 2004;16(6):690-699.

(22) Montero-Odasso M, Levinson P, Gore B, Epid D, Tremblay L, Bergman H. A flowchart system to improve fall data documentation in a long-term care institution: a pilot study. J Am Med Dir Assoc 2007;8(5):300-306.

(23) Shostack GL. Understanding services through blueprinting. In: Swartz TA, Bowen DE, Brown SW, editors. Advances in Services Marketing and Management.Greenwich, Conn.: JAI Press; 1992. 75-90.

(24) Kingman-Brundage J. The ABC's of service blueprinting. In: Bitner MJ, Crosby LA, editors. Designing Winning Service Strategies.Chicago, Illinois: American Marketing Association; 1989. 30-33.

(25) Holdford DA, Kennedy DT. Service blueprint as a tool for designing innovative pharmaceutical services. Journal of the American Pharmaceutical Association 39[Jul-Aug], 545-552. 1999.

(26) Robert J, Xiangyu K. The customer experience: a road-map for improvement. Managing Service Quality 2011;21(1):5-24.

(27) David WN, Pine II BJ. Using the customer journey to road test and refine the business model. Strategy & Leadership 2013;41(2):12-17.

(28) Clatworthy S. Service Innovation Through Touch-points: Development of an Innovation Toolkit for the First Stages of New Service Development. International Journal of Design 2011;5(2).

Chapter Questions

1. What approach to service design is most common in your work setting— the production line or empowerment approach? Explain your answer.

2. Could a production line approach to service design be consistent with the provision of medication therapy management? Why or why not?

3. How might service scripts be used in your pharmacy school to learn important skills? What skills should be learned through service scripts? When would a script not work?

4. How might pharmacists make some of their backstage performances more visible to patients and other customers?

Activities

1. Develop a script for what to say or do in one of the following service situations. Each person must choose a different situation. If it is useful in your practice setting, you may develop scripts for situations not listed here.

Dispensing error

Situation requiring a physician to change a prescribed therapy

Nonformulary prescription

Need for prior authorization

Nursing administration error

Patient complaint about the price of a prescription

Drug incompatibility

Physician prescribing error

Drug allergy

Drug interaction

Service mistake (e.g., overcharge)

Negotiation with co-workers over work schedules

Difficult patient counseling situation

Patient with renal insufficiency

Patient with hepatic insufficiency

Hostile customer

2. Choose a service with which you are familiar and develop a service blueprint for it (e.g., dispensing a prescription). Identify activities that are hidden from the patient or other customer (e.g., nurse) and those that provide evidence for quality from the patient's viewpoint.

PART **IV**

Consumer Behavior

CHAPTER **10**

CONSUMERS' EVALUATION OF SERVICES

Objectives

After studying this chapter, the reader should be able to

- o   Define the key terms including: satisfaction, dissatisfaction, service quality, value, expectations, technical quality, and functional quality
- o   Discuss why pharmacists should care about patient perceptions of service
- o   List the 10 dimensions of service quality that patients use to evaluate pharmaceutical services
- o   Describe the two dimensions of service quality most important in determining overall perceptions of service
- o   Compare and contrast affective loyalty and behavioral loyalty
- o   Explain why dissatisfaction is more important than satisfaction in determining patient perceptions of service
- o   Suggest things pharmacists can do to understand and influence patient perception of services

This chapter discusses how consumers evaluate services—pharmacist services in particular. It explains what determines satisfaction and perceptions of service quality. Important dimensions of service and their impact on overall assessments of service are also discussed. Finally, the chapter describes the link between patient perceptions of service and patient behavior.

MARKETING IN ACTION

What does the old guy have that I don't?

The young pharmacist, Scott, could not understand what made patients tick. Here he was - the most clinically competent employee in the pharmacy. But when patients came to the pharmacy, they always asked for Julius.

Julius was an older pharmacist who was a nice guy but not nearly as knowledgeable as Scott about pharmacy therapeutics and medications. It annoyed Scott that Julius would waste time chatting with patients about family members, the weather, and other trivial issues instead of filling prescriptions.

Scott could fill prescriptions in half the time that Julius took, but the patients continued to prefer Julius over him. Scott was proud about how he dealt with patients quickly and professionally. In fact, he always counseled the patients he served, whether or not they wanted counseling.

Still, the patients continued to ask for Julius.

SATISFACTION

Satisfaction results when a customer evaluates a purchase he or she has made and concludes that the product or service meets or exceeds expectations.[1] *Dissatisfaction* results when it fails to meet expectations. Various factors contribute to satisfaction or dissatisfaction with pharmacy service experiences (Figure 10-1).

Figure 10-1: Antecedents and Consequences of Customer Satisfaction

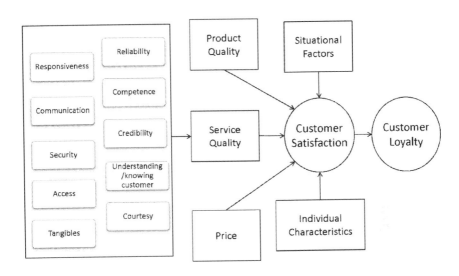

Satisfaction with a pharmacy visit may be influenced by the responsiveness of the pharmacist to the needs of the patient (i.e., service quality), perceptions of how the drug worked (i.e., product quality), and the price paid (i.e., value). Satisfaction is also influenced by factors beyond the marketer's control. Both the situation in which the service is provided and the characteristics of the person assessing the service affect satisfaction. The weather or traffic on the way to the pharmacy can influence a patient's evaluation, as can personal factors like fatigue or irritability.

The comparison of performance with expectations is called the process of *expectancy disconfirmation*[2] (Figure 10-2). Disconfirmation of expectations can be positive or negative. Negative disconfirmation occurs when performance does not meet expectations; the consumer is dissatisfied.

When performance meets expectations, confirmation occurs; the consumer is either mildly satisfied or not dissatisfied. Positive disconfirmation occurs when performance exceeds expectations; the consumer is satisfied. *"Customer delight"*[3] occurs when the consumer is extremely satisfied as a result of some unexpected, pleasant surprise (e.g., a pharmacist who goes out of the way to help solve a patient problem).

Figure 10-2 Results of comparing perceived service performance with expectations

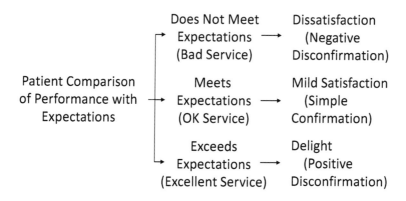

As an example of disconfirmation, consider a woman who visits a pharmacy with her 7-year-old daughter to fill a prescription for the child's ear infection. In the past, the girl has been very finicky about taking medications. Administering each dose has been a major battle between the mother and the child. In addition, the mother is anxious about the girl's health, and the illness has disrupted the whole family's daily routine.

If the pharmacist fills the prescription quickly and accurately, the mother's expectations are met and she is mildly satisfied with the service. The mother's anxiety about her finicky child has not been resolved, but her minimal expectation of receiving the drug in a timely manner has been met. If the mother's minimal expectation is not met (e.g., the pharmacist makes the mother wait too long or is unintentionally rude), negative disconfirmation occurs and the mother is dissatisfied.

But the pharmacist does more than what is minimally expected. He speaks directly to the girl in a pleasant and serious manner. Crouching down to her eye level, he tells the girl about the antibiotic and the importance of taking it. The girl is allowed to choose from several flavorings (bubblegum, grape, and cherry). The pharmacist adds the girl's choice (bubblegum) and water to the powdered drug and then asks the girl to help shake the ingredients in the bottle. The pharmacist tells the girl that it is her responsibility to shake the medicine before every dose; otherwise, the medicine will not work. With great seriousness and commitment, the girl shakes the bottle and promises to follow the pharmacist's directions.

The mother is delighted, because she has just seen a pharmacist persuade her finicky child to take the medication. The pharmacy has just gained a loyal customer, because the pharmacist went out of the way to help.

Consumer satisfaction is important to marketers and service providers for several reasons. Satisfaction with businesses has been shown to increase repeat purchasing intentions and behaviors.[2, 4] Consumers who are satisfied are more likely to say good things to friends and family members and less likely to complain to them.[5] Positive word of mouth can often be more effective in attracting new customers than most forms of advertising and promotion.

Furthermore, businesses that continually satisfy customers with quality services are more profitable, on average. Satisfaction has been associated with increased market share, the ability to charge customers higher prices, higher return on investment, and profitability.[6]

EXPECTATIONS

It is clear from the previous discussion that expectations about service delivery and outcome are an important aspect of satisfaction. Consumers' evaluation of services is affected by their expectations about performance. Consumers who have low expectations are easy to please, and those with high expectations are more likely to be disappointed.

Consumer expectations of services have upper and lower boundaries: minimally acceptable and most desired[7] (i.e., adequate for minimal satisfaction and likely to produce customer delight, respectively). Services that fall between minimally acceptable and most desired are in the zone of tolerance[8] (Figure 10-3). Service in the zone of tolerance is perceived as neither excellent nor bad. It is merely adequate and causes only mild satisfaction. Services that consistently fall within the zone of tolerance neither attract customers nor drive them away.

Merely adequate services provide no competitive advantage to businesses. When service is only adequate, competitive advantage must come from other sources, such as merchandise, location, price, or other elements of the marketing mix. Pharmacists who merely meet patient expectations provide the minimum performance necessary to satisfy patients. Meeting expectations is fine in an environment without competition. It generates mildly positive feelings about the pharmacist and keeps the patient loyal—as long as no competitor offers anything better.

Figure 10-3 Zone of tolerance for services

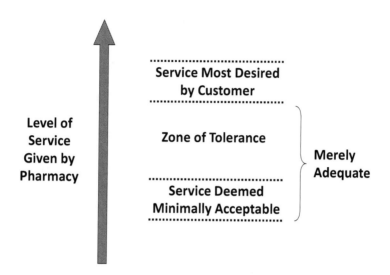

PERCEIVED VALUE AND SERVICE QUALITY

Also related to consumers' perceptions of service are perceived value and service quality. *Perceived value* is the consumer's overall assessment of utility, based on comparing what is received with what was spent in dollars, time, and effort.[7] In other words, value refers to a consumer's perception of the tradeoff between benefits and costs. A patient's perception of the value of pharmacy services depends on the quality of those services, the benefits resulting from that quality, and the amount of money, time, and effort spent in receiving those benefits.

Service quality refers to customer perceptions of the quality of services over time. It is closely related to, yet distinct from, satisfaction.[9] Satisfaction refers to customer perceptions not only of the quality of services but also of products, price, and other non-service-related factors. Service quality can be described as satisfaction with the quality of service provided.

Service Elements Assessed by Consumers

Some services can be difficult to assess. When you go to an auto mechanic, it is difficult to know whether the mechanic performed all the services he claims to have performed. In most cases, you have to take the mechanic's word that he replaced a part or changed a fluid.

Similarly, the quality of a pharmacist's work in filling a prescription can be difficult to assess, because patients cannot evaluate factors such as the accuracy of record keeping or the clinical expertise of the pharmacist. Some aspects of pharmacy service can be evaluated only after consumption (e.g., a pharmacist's recommendation for a nonprescription headache medication).

Some attributes can be identified and evaluated before choosing or consuming a service. A pharmacy's location is one such attribute because the consumer can evaluate it by finding it on a map or driving past it. Other attributes can only be evaluated after purchase or use; pain relief from a recommended drug and the friendliness of pharmacy personnel are examples. Finally, some attributes can never be accurately assessed by consumers. Most technical services provided by pharmacists, cannot be evaluated even after experiencing them because patients do not have the knowledge or expertise to evaluate them. Many medications must be used for long periods of time before their effects can be seen, and even then it may be uncertain whether the patient's health outcome was the result of a particular therapy.

In general, medical services are difficult to assess. Like all services, they are intangible, inconsistent, and inseparable. Moreover, the practice of medicine is complex and requires substantial training and education. Most patients feel uncomfortable judging the more technical aspects of medical care.

For these reasons, patients are likely to assess health care services on attributes they can evaluate.[10, 11] Patient satisfaction with physician visits is likely to be determined more by the amount of time the physician spends with the patient than by the technical aspects of care. In choosing pharmacies, patients rely on nontechnical aspects of care like convenience and friendly service.[12, 13]

Technical and Functional Quality

The quality of services has both technical and functional components.[10, 14] *Technical quality* refers to the end result of services (i.e., outcomes). Elements of pharmacist services that affect technical quality are those activities that result in receiving the right drug and maximizing the appropriateness of drug use (e.g., reviewing the patient medication profile, therapeutic monitoring, and counseling). *Functional quality* refers to the process in which services are provided (e.g., responsive, reliable).

Patients judge pharmacy service quality on the basis of their perceptions of both the technical and functional components,[10] but functional quality plays a greater role. Although a positive outcome of pharmacy service is always desired, patients tend to rate their pharmacists on the basis of their social interactions rather than their technical skills. Patients do not have the expertise or information necessary to evaluate the technical quality of health care. Instead, they consider how personable a pharmacist is or how neatly she is dressed. In fact, a technically competent pharmacist with poor interpersonal skills may be rated lower by patients than a less competent pharmacist with good interpersonal capabilities.

> The customer's perception is your reality.
>
> -Kate Zabriskie, Service Training Expert

Dimensions of Service

Marketers refer to 10 generic dimensions that are important in consumers' evaluation of service (Table 10-1).[15] These dimensions primarily address functional quality. Although any of the 10 dimensions can determine a consumer's judgment of service, some dimensions are more important than others. Reliability is considered the most important driver of overall perception of services.[9, 16] Reliability addresses the question, "Are services provided accurately and dependably?" It also indirectly relates to other service dimensions such as credibility (i.e., Will the pharmacist keep his promises?) and competence (i.e., Is the pharmacist competent to provide services without mistakes?).

Reliability is a core element of value provided by pharmacists. A pharmacist's work is expected to be error free; otherwise, a patient could be injured or even killed. Reliability is also the foundation for credibility and trust. A pharmacist who is not dependable or cannot be expected to keep promises will not be able to maintain the trust of customers.

The second most important dimension driving consumers' evaluation of service is responsiveness.[9,16] Responsiveness encompasses both willingness and capability to respond to customers in a timely manner. A responsive pharmacist is attentive to patients' requests for assistance, questions about the location of pharmacy merchandise, and complaints about services. Even when a pharmacist cannot solve a patient's problem, it is essential that the pharmacist be perceived as willing to do so. Responsiveness also refers to the perceived speed of service. A patient who has to wait for prescriptions or counseling about medications typically rates responsiveness as low.

Other dimensions of service quality can determine whether a consumer will patronize a business. Credibility is essential in health care. Pharmacists make recommendations that affect a patient's health and daily activities. Those recommendations must inspire patients' trust and confidence. Communication is necessary to help patients understand how to take their medications and to clear up misunderstandings about issues such as pricing. The risk associated with prescription drugs makes security an important dimension. Even the physical appearance of facilities and personnel (tangibles) sends a message of competence and quality to patients. The relative importance of individual dimensions in the evaluation of a service experience depends in part on the consumer and the circumstances of the visit. A pharmacy's appearance may be important for someone who is shopping for birthday cards but irrelevant for a quick visit to purchase soda or snacks.

To maximize patient assessments of service quality, pharmacists should focus on being reliable first and responsive second. This means putting a system in place in which errors do not occur, service is timely, and employees care about serving the patient. When these dimensions of service are maintained at a consistently high level, pharmacists can work on the other dimensions of service.

Table 10-1 Dimensions of Service Quality

Tangibles: The appearance of physical facilities and personnel. The tools or equipment used to provide the service. Written information provided as part of the service.

Reliability: Performing the service correctly the first time. Honoring promises through accurate billing, precise record keeping, and performance of the service when promised.

Responsiveness: Willingness and ability to provide prompt service. Involves timeliness of service.

Communication: Explaining service to customers in language they can understand. Involves explaining the service itself, describing how much it will cost, explaining the tradeoffs between service and cost, and assuring the customer that the problem will be resolved.

Credibility: Trustworthiness, believability, and honesty of customer-contact personnel and company.

Security: Freedom from danger, risk, and doubt. Involves physical safety (e.g., Will following the pharmacist's directions cause me harm?), financial security (e.g., Will I be able to pay for my drugs?), and confidentiality of transactions (e.g., Will the other customers hear about my physical ailments?).

Competence: Customer-contact personnel's possession of the required skills and knowledge to perform the service.

Understanding/knowing the customer: Involves learning a customer's specific requirements, providing individualized attention, and recognizing a regular customer.

Access: Involves approachability and ease of contact. Includes accessibility by telephone, convenient operating hours and location, and reasonable waiting time for service.

Courtesy: Politeness, respect, consideration, and friendliness of customer-contact personnel. Includes clean and neat appearance of customer-contact personnel.

Source: Reference 15

Customer Loyalty

Customers' satisfaction and perception of service quality are important because they relate to measures of business performance, including profitability. Consumer perceptions of service are frequently used as a proxy measure for consumer behavior and business profitability.

One problem with using satisfaction as the sole outcome measure of services is that the link between satisfaction and patronage tends to be weak and inconsistent. Even when satisfied, consumers often switch to other service providers. Research shows that between 65% and 85% of consumers who report being satisfied or very satisfied with their former service provider will switch to other providers.[17] Even consumers who are considered loyal continue to do business with other providers.[18] This suggests that consumer satisfaction alone may be a poor predictor of profitability.

Thus, when given freedom of choice, a satisfied patient of a community pharmacy may decide to visit a competing pharmacy just out of curiosity or because of a discount on a transferred prescription. Even when content, people may investigate other providers for better service and price offers, particularly if there is no perception of risk or hassle involved.[19] Restrictions on the freedom to choose pharmacies can further cloud the link between satisfaction and patronage. When a pharmacy benefit manager restricts patients to a limited network of pharmacies, patients may be dissatisfied with the network pharmacies but continue to use them to avoid paying for their drugs out of pocket. In rural areas, dissatisfied patients may continue to patronize a pharmacy if competing pharmacies are too far away. In these cases, satisfaction may have little relationship to patient patronage and thus profitability.

Businesses have begun to emphasize the importance of customer loyalty, as well as satisfaction. *Customer loyalty* is defined as continual patronage of a service provider, and it is claimed to be the single most important determinant of long-term financial performance.[20]

Loyal customers lead to increased profitability and productivity because they are more likely to repurchase goods and services and to repurchase in greater quantity, and they cost less to retain.[6, 20, 21] Customer loyalty involves positive feelings toward an organization as well as ongoing patronage. Thus, loyalty has both an affective and a behavioral component. When consumers speak highly of a business or express a preference over competitors, this is *affective loyalty*. People who are delighted with a business express affective loyalty. When consumers increase purchases of goods and services or willingly pay a premium price, this is *behavioral loyalty*. Consumers who have high levels of affective loyalty are also likely to demonstrate high levels of behavioral loyalty.[6, 20, 21]

> There is a big difference between a satisfied customer and a loyal customer.
>
> - Shep Hyken, Customer Service Expert

SATISFACTION AND BEHAVIORAL LOYALTY

The relationship between consumer satisfaction and behavioral loyalty often is not linear. Improvements in consumer satisfaction are not necessarily associated with equivalent changes in consumer loyalty. The relationship between satisfaction and behavioral loyalty depends in part on a consumer's ability to freely move from one service provider to another.[22] If consumers are free to choose, dissatisfaction will lead to decreased loyalty. But consumers' ability to respond to dissatisfaction may be restricted by a lack of competitors or by contractual limitations of prescription insurance plans.

Thus, in noncompetitive environments, such as rural areas underserved by pharmacists, locales where patients do not have freedom of pharmacy choice because of managed care restrictions, and communities where a pharmacy may be the only provider offering a unique, highly desired service, there is much less sensitivity to changes in patient satisfaction. Only when consumers become extremely dissatisfied will substantial defections to competitors occur.

In noncompetitive environments, relationships with a business may be based on some barrier to leaving that relationship, not on a continued desire to maintain the relationship. For example, many people only stay with specific cable TV companies or mobile phone providers because there are no better options -- not because they are satisfied. Dissatisfied consumers maintain a relationship only as long as they must. Once the barriers that prevent free choice are removed, the consumer very likely will leave that service provider.

Effect of Dissatisfaction

Negative experiences with pharmacy service are likely to have a greater impact on overall patient satisfaction than positive service experiences. Providing excellent service is important in exceeding patient expectations, but it is more important not to dissatisfy patients with poor service experiences.[23] When a prescription is filled 10 minutes faster than promised or expected, this has a positive but limited effect on overall patient satisfaction. Waiting 10 minutes longer than expected for a prescription is likely to have a disproportionately greater negative effect on overall satisfaction.

The reason is that consumers pay more attention to bad service than to good service and are more likely to remember bad service experiences.[23] Consumers expect to receive good service in most cases. If prescriptions are dispensed correctly, patients will only be "not dissatisfied," because error-free dispensing is taken for granted. But when expectations of good service are not met, patients may feel unfairly treated and take action in response.

That action might include discontinuing business with the service provider or complaining to others. Consumers are more likely to complain to others about bad service than to make positive comments about good service. Consumers tell an average of 5 other people when they receive good service, whereas they tell 9 to 11 others when they receive bad service.[24] Because consumers attach more significance to negative service experiences, a highly satisfied consumer can quickly become a highly dissatisfied consumer.

MARKETING IN ACTION

United Breaks Guitars

"United Breaks Guitars" is a YouTube hit that recently exceeded 14.5 million views. The video is a combination protest song and reenactment of a trip that Canadian musician Dave Carroll and his band, Sons of Maxwell had on a United Airlines Flight leaving from Chicago's O'Hare International Airport. The song and video became a public relations debacle for the airline.

According to the video and song, Carroll said his guitar was broken while in United Airlines' custody. He reported that he was sitting in his seat on the plane during a layover on a flight from Halifax to Omaha, Nebraska. One of his fellow passengers said that baggage handlers at Chicago's O'Hare were throwing guitars around on the tarmac. After arriving in Omaha, he discovered that his $3,500 Taylor guitar was severely damaged. Carroll reportedly:

1. alerted three employees who showed indifference to his concerns

2. Filed a claim with United Airlines who informed him that he was ineligible for compensation because he had failed to make the claim within its

stipulated "standard 24-hour timeframe"

3.   spent nine months trying to negotiate with United to compensate him for the damage

In complete frustration, Carroll decided to write a song and create a music video about his experience. The video recreates his experience and the unresponsiveness of United employees and management. The lyrics include verses like:

You broke it, you should fix it
You're liable, just admit it
I should've flown with someone else
Or gone by car

And the refrain goes:

United...

(United...)

You broke my Taylor Guitar

United...

(United...)

Some big help you are

Numerous national media outlets reported on the story and of the nerve struck by the song's instant success. No amount of spin or damage control by United Airlines was able to undo the damage done to its image. Since the incident, Carroll has been in favorite speaker at meetings (including NCPA's 2014 Annual Convention and Trade Exposition) about customer service.

IMPROVING PATIENT PERCEPTIONS OF SERVICE

Assessing Perceptions of Service

There are many ways for pharmacists to assess patient perceptions of service. They differ in complexity, cost, and the degree to which they inconvenience the patient. The choice of technique depends on the purpose of the feedback, the budget, and the available time.

The key to making patient feedback pay off is to develop a tracking system that permits analysis and action. Patient responses that are simply filed away cannot be used to improve service. Furthermore, to obtain usable recommendations for improving service, the right questions need to be asked, in a way that effectively elicits patient comments. The following are common in pharmacies

- Observation - Observing patient interactions with pharmacists and technicians can identify service problems. Observation can identify unproductive practices, length of time spent in various activities, and customer responses.

- Employee feedback - Employees know many of the problems within service systems and can suggest solutions. They can also assess the quality of internal marketing initiatives. Employee feedback should be solicited with any service venture.

- Patient complaints - Patient complaints can help identify which aspects of service are most irritating. Complaints may indicate just the tip of the iceberg and reveal a serious service problem. Service recovery strategies should be developed to deal with complaints. Complaints on social media sites like Yelp can help identify areas needing improvement.

- Patient interviews - Patients can be interviewed formally or casually about their assessments of pharmacist services. Most good pharmacists ask patients how they are doing and how they can improve.

- Patient surveys - Surveys can solicit patient feedback about service while experiences are still fresh in the patient's mind. The shorter and more accessible the survey, the better.

- Critical incident surveys - Critical incident surveys are designed to identify particularly good and bad services. Patients are asked to describe the details of service incidents that stand out in their minds (e.g., "Describe a particularly good or bad experience you had with a pharmacist").

- Focus groups - Focus groups are gatherings of patients who are invited to discuss issues of importance. They can be used to solicit quick, informal insight into service problems.

- Mystery Shoppers - Mystery, or secret, shoppers are often used to supplement patient feedback. They provide analysis of specific service features that patient feedback may overlook. A mystery shopper who visits a pharmacy typically has a checklist for assessing aspects of service such as whether the pharmacist greeted the patient, offered to counsel about the medications, was friendly and helpful, checked the patient profile, and completed other required tasks. Most patients are not able to assess the service experience as critically or in as much detail as trained and observant mystery shoppers can.

o   Sales figures - Sales figures are the ultimate measure of patient satisfaction. Patient perceptions of service should be linked to total sales, repeat sales, and other sales figures to identify which measures are most predictive of sales.

Measuring Loyalty

Loyalty should be measured, since it is an important indicator of profitability. Measures of loyalty include intention to repurchase, actual repurchase, and positive word-of-mouth recommendations.[20] It is easy and convenient to ask consumers about intentions to repurchase a product or service. Intention-to-repurchase measures are strong indicators of future behavior, but they generally overstate the probability of repurchase.[20] People who report that they intend to purchase do not always do so. Usually this overstatement is not a significant problem, because the extent of overstatement is consistent. Adjustments can be made to correct for the overstatement, resulting in relatively accurate predictions.[20]

Sales data provide information about actual repurchase behavior, including how recently, how frequently, and how long repurchases have occurred and the amounts of these purchases. These measurements can be used to determine change resulting from marketing interventions. The data are easy to gather from computer databases. In pharmacy firms, repurchase data might include the percentage of patients who refill prescriptions or transfer prescriptions to other pharmacies.

Consumer referrals and positive word-of-mouth recommendations are associated with short-term and long-term judgments about purchasing behavior.[20] Such referrals and recommendations indicate the strength of feelings about services (i.e., affective loyalty); they are less directly linked to actual purchase behavior. When all forms of loyalty measures are used together, they can provide a comprehensive picture of consumer loyalty and can supplement satisfaction data.

Prioritizing Service Quality Initiatives

Pharmacists have limited resources to improve the quality of their services, so they need to select marketing approaches that optimize patient loyalty. It often pays for pharmacists to focus on service deficiencies to reduce dissatisfaction, rather than trying to increase satisfaction. To reduce the number of patients dissatisfied with a pharmacy organization, several strategies can be used.

First, target patients who can be best satisfied by the pharmacy. Some individuals become dissatisfied with services not through the fault of the program, but because they are just a poor match for what the program offers. Patient selection is critical for ensuring that patient expectations match the services being provided.

Also, educate patients about what to expect. When expectations are unreasonable, open communication with the patient can sometimes adjust expectations.

Prevent service-related failures from occurring in the first place. This requires a service system that continually seeks to root out causes of failure and correct them.

Practice service recovery once a service failure has occurred. Pharmacies need to have a plan in place for use when failures occur.

SUMMARY

Patients base their evaluations of pharmacy services on a complex mix of expectations and perceptions. Positive perceptions are associated with patient loyalty, positive word-of-mouth recommendations, and profitability.

Pharmacists who want to maximize their impact on patient perceptions should focus on specific aspects of their services. They should attempt to make their service as reliable and responsive as possible, and to minimize negative service experiences. Finally, pharmacists should monitor patient perceptions of service to identify ways of improving the services they provide.

Reference List

(1) Szymanski DM, Henard DH. Customer satisfaction: A meta-analysis of the empirical evidence. *Journal of the Academy of Marketing Science* 2001;29(1):16-35.

(2) Oliver RL. A cognitive model of the antecedents and consequences of satisfaction decisions. *Journal of Marketing Research* 1980;460-469.

(3) Schneider B, Bowen DE. Understanding customer delight and outrage. *Sloan Management Review* 1999;41(1):35-+.

(4) Oliver RL. *Satisfaction: A behavioral perspective on the consumer*. ME sharpe; 2010.

(5) Anderson EW. Customer satisfaction and word of mouth. *Journal of Service Research* 1998;1(1):5-17.

(6) Zeithaml VA, Berry LL, Parasuraman A. The behavioral consequences of service quality. *Journal of Marketing* 1996;60(2):31-46.

(7) Zeithaml VA, MJ. B. *Services Marketing*. 1st ed. New York: McGraw-Hill Companies Inc.; 1996.

(8) Zeithaml VA, Berry LL, Parasuraman A. The nature and determinants of customer expectations of service. *Journal of the Academy of Marketing Science* 1993;21(1):1-12.

(9) Parasuraman A, Zeithaml V, Berry L. SERVQUAL: A multi item scale for measuring consumer perception of service quality. *J Retailing* 1988;64(Spring):12-40.

(10) Holdford D, Schulz R. Effect of technical and functional quality on patient perceptions of pharmaceutical service quality. Pharmaceutical Research 16[Sep], 1344-1351. 1999.

(11) Chang JT, Hays RD, Shekelle PG et al. Patients' global ratings of their health care are not associated with the technical quality of their care. *Annals of Internal Medicine* 2006;144(9):665-672.

(12) Patterson BJ, Doucette WR, Urmie JM, McDonough RP. Exploring relationships among pharmacy service use, patronage motives, and patient satisfaction. *J Am Pharm Assoc (2003)* 2013;53(4):382-389.

(13) Franic DM, Haddock SM, Tucker LT, Wooten N. Pharmacy patronage: identifying key factors in the decision making process using the determinant attribute approach. *J Am Pharm Assoc (2003)* 2008;48(1):71-85.

(14) Gronroos C. *Service Marketing and Management*. Lexington, MA.: Lexington Books; 1990.

(15) Parasuraman A, Zeithaml V, Berry L. A conceptual model of service quality and its implications for future research. *Journal of Marketing or J Marketing* 1985;49(Fall):41-50.

(16) Parasuraman A ZVBL. Refinement and reassessment of the SERVQUAL scale. *Journal of Retailing* 1991;67(4):420-450.

(17) Reichheld Ff. Loyalty-Based Management. *Harvard Business Review* 1993;71(2):64-73.

(18) O'Malley L. Can loyalty schemes really build loyalty? *Marketing Intelligence & Planning* 1998;16(1):47-55.

(19) Dowling GR, Uncles M. Do customer loyalty programs really work? *Sloan Management Review* 1997;38(4):71-81.

(20) Jones To, Sasser We. Why Satisfied Customers Defect. *Harvard Business Review* 1995;73(6):88-92.

(21) Reichheld FE. Customer service on British Airways. *Harvard Business Review* 1996;74(1):166.

(22) Heskett Jl, Jones To, Loveman Gw, Sasser We, Schlesinger La. Putting The Service-Profit Chain To Work. *Harvard Business Review* 1994;72(2):164-174.

(23) Mittal V, Ross WT, Baldasare PM. The asymmetric impact of negative and positive attribute-level performance on overall satisfaction and repurchase intentions. *Journal of Marketing* 1998;62(1):33-47.

(24) [Anon]. The service profit chain - Heskett,JL, Sasser,WE, Schlesinger,LA. *Sloan Management Review* 1997;38(3):107.

Chapter Questions

1. Discuss the differences between being satisfied, dissatisfied, and delighted with services.

2. Is it necessary for patients to be satisfied with their health care? Should pharmacists attempt to achieve 100% patient satisfaction? Explain your answer.

3. How might patient expectations influence perceptions of pharmacist performance? What determines patient expectations of pharmacist services? In what situations might pharmacists want to lower patient expectations?

4. Describe the relationship between patient satisfaction and loyalty to the pharmacy.

5. Which of the 10 dimensions of service quality are most important in patients' overall perception of pharmacist services? In your opinion, which ones are least important?

6. How might patients and pharmacists differ in their perceptions of the quality of pharmacy services? Who would be the most critical of the services, and why?

7. How does functional quality influence the technical quality of pharmacy services?

CONSUMER BEHAVIOR

> "All human actions have one or more of these seven causes: chance, nature, compulsions, habit, reason, passion and desire."
>
> - Aristotle

Understanding the behavior of consumers is a fundamental requirement for marketing pharmacy products and pharmacist services. Good marketers realize how and why consumers make decisions about the purchase and use of drugs. Knowledge about consumer behavior is essential in setting prices, merchandising, advertising, designing services, and other marketing activities.

Decision-making in health care differs from consumer decisions about purchasing nonhealth products and services in many situations. In health care, the consumer (i.e., the patient) frequently does not choose the treatment to be consumed (e.g., the drug). Often, that decision is left to the physician or other health care professional. Health care is also unique because patients usually pay directly only a fraction of the cost. Most costs are paid by third-party payers such as insurance companies, employers, and the government. These third-party payers exert significant influence on consumer decisions.

Detailed discussion of the many decision makers in health care is beyond the scope of this book. This chapter focuses on decision-making by patients as consumers. Understanding patient decision-making is important for pharmacists because of the large number of consumer-generated pharmacy transactions (e.g., nonprescription and herbal products, general merchandise) and the expanding role of consumers in health care choices.

CONSUMER DECISIONS

Consumers make decisions to fulfill their unmet needs and wants. A patient goes to a pharmacy to satisfy some desire (e.g., treat a cold). The patient's decision about how to fulfill that desire is influenced by a variety of personal, social, and economic factors, such as perceptions of risk and recommendations from friends. The following paragraphs describe three frameworks for understanding consumer behavior.

Economic man. Much of what marketers know about consumer behavior originates from economics. Economic understanding of consumer behavior is based in part on the assumptions that (1) people are rational in their behavior, (2) they attempt to maximize personal satisfaction through exchange, (3) they possess complete information on available alternatives, and (4) they use that information to make a choice. The model of economic man is useful in identifying behaviors relating to price, consumer income, quality, and consumer tastes. From economics, we know that demand for a drug is positively associated with low prices for the drug, high prices for drug substitutes, high consumer income, consumer tastes, and the quality of the drug and accompanying service.

However, economics makes many assumptions about consumers that are not borne out in real life. Often, consumers make choices irrationally (i.e., they act in ways that seem contrary to their best interests) and lack or ignore information that could be used in making choices.[1, 2] Furthermore, the classic economic man framework does not consider many cultural, social, and psychological influences on demand. The following are some examples of behavior that is inconsistent with economic principles:

- o Pay-for-performance programs (P4P). P4P programs offer monetary rewards to motivate behaviors of health care providers to improve the quality of care. Research shows that pay-for-performance programs often backfire by undermining motivation and worsening performance.[3] Extrinsic rewards often crowd out intrinsic desires to do the right thing and encourage cheating and gaming the rewards system.

- o Placebo effect. It is well known that placebos can reduce pain. However, the price of placebos should have no effect on pain relief according to classical economics. That would be irrational. Nevertheless, subjects who received electric shocks had greater relief from placebo pills that were priced at $2.50 per pill than from placebos priced at $0.10 per pill.[4] This means that higher priced medications can have a greater placebo effect.

- o Framing the question. When people are presented with two health care choices (Option A where 200 out of 600 patients will be saved and Option B where 400 out of 600 patients will die), three quarters of people will choose Option A.[1] Classical economics confidently predicts that equal numbers will choose A and B because both result in 200 patients living and 600 patients dying. However, framing Option A as "saving" patients is perceived as the less risky option.

Social influences. Much of consumer behavior is influenced by our interactions with others. From birth, humans are influenced by subtle pressures that form our desires and actions. These pressures can emanate from social norms established by peer groups, reference groups, family, and social class. Much of our understanding of drug use is founded on social theories. Social networks are associated with numerous health related behaviors including smoking,[5] obesity,[6] and alcohol use.[7]

Personal influences. Each person is driven by a variety of desires and pressures that influence behavior. Complex psychological processes occur that are difficult for others to see but crucial to how we act. Consumer behavior is influenced by our personality, values, beliefs, and attitudes. As might be expected, much of what we know about personal influences comes from the field of psychology.

Marketers draw from these frameworks and many others to understand consumer behavior. Economics and social sciences provide the foundation of most marketing theory and practices. As a result, many processes in pharmaceutical marketing originate from other disciplines.

For example, interventions to improve patient adherence to drug regimens is largely based on our understanding of economic, social, and psychological behavior. Economics has an obvious effect when patients have to pay all or a portion of the costs of the medications they consume. Social and demographic variables (age, sex, marital status, size of household, social class, attitudes of peers and family members) affect compliance in ways that may be hard to predict. Psychological and cognitive influences include the patient's knowledge, mental capability, and beliefs about medicine, self-efficacy, and previous experiences. Nonadherence is a complex issue that requires sophisticated interventions by providers, who must integrate their knowledge of disease, therapies, and patient behaviors.

MARKETING IN ACTION

Drug Store Visits Begin at the Doctor's Office

A recent study highlights the important link between physicians and pharmacists.[8] It found that visits to the physician office are often followed by a pharmacy visits. Six out of ten people who visited their physician also visited a pharmacy that same day. For those with prescriptions, 95% visited a pharmacy.

The study polled patients in doctor's office waiting rooms about attitudes and preferences for managing their health, and how pharmacies were utilized as a health resource. They found that that consumers were more likely to shop at chain pharmacies and mass merchandisers and that store location/convenience is still a key driver for their pharmacy selection.

Visitors to physician office differ from the general population because they visit pharmacies more often (up 47%), fill more prescriptions (up 48%) and spend more time overall in stores during a pharmacy visit (up 39%) than the average consumer. Patients under a physician's care can even be called "drug store super shoppers,"

Super shoppers fall into different categories including:

- o "Wellness Seekers" - proactive about their health, regular visitors to the physician, and seeking healthy lifestyle options
- o "Aging Americans" - looking to push back the ravages of medical conditions related to aging and manage their chronic and acute conditions
- o "Episodic Sufferers" - looking to treat acute conditions with prescriptions or over-the-counter medications

Super shopper spending at pharmacies comes from the greater number of prescriptions filled and additional sales from non-pharmacy merchandise across the store. Seven-in-ten from this group of shoppers reported that they purchase one or more over-the-counter medications (including vitamins) during an average trip to the pharmacy, and six-in-ten purchase personal hygiene products.

The link between physician visits and drug store sales support shopper marketing strategies like one-stop shopping. Pharmacy chains continue to expand their selection of products, including household items, food and beverages and more to capture additional sales.

Source: Reference [8]

CONSUMER PURCHASE SITUATIONS

Consumer decisions fall into two categories: new and repeat decisions (Figure 11-1). The first visit to a pharmacy or the choice of a new cough and cold preparation would be a new decision. A visit to a pharmacy to refill a prescription or buy more nonprescription pain medication would be a repeat decision.

New decisions range from the complex to the simple. Complex decisions tend to involve extended problem solving and substantial consideration and effort by the consumer. Major health care decisions, such as a decision to undergo surgery, typically require extended problem solving. Limited problem solving is used for simple problems that can be handled without much mental effort. Impulse purchases (i.e., unplanned, spur-of-the-moment reactions to a presented product) are the least complex form of problem solving.

Figure 11-1 Types of Consumer Decisions

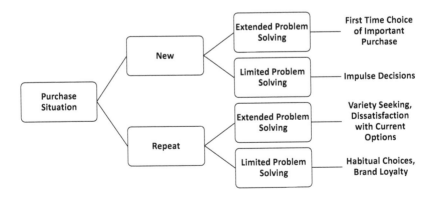

Repeat decisions also range from the complex to the simple, and they account for many consumer and health care decisions. Typically, repeat decisions require less contemplation than new decisions and can be handled with limited problem solving. Consumers use experience gained from previous decisions to simplify the purchase process. Patients often remain loyal to nonprescription cough and cold medications because they remember that previous use brought them relief. Rather than carefully weigh each alternative, the consumer simply chooses the brand that worked the last time.

Consumers' use of extended or limited problem solving depends on a variety of factors. Extended problem solving occurs more often with new, high-risk, and complex problems. It is more likely to be used by someone who is engaged in a first-time search for a drug to treat a severe, multisymptom cold than by someone in search of a frequently purchased headache medication. Extended problem solving is also more likely when the consumer has time for and interest in the decision. Busy consumers often do not have the luxury of time for detailed analysis of the options.

The degree to which patients engage in problem solving has important implications for pharmacists. Patients who engage in extended problem solving want information and are more likely to pay attention to longer, more thoughtful messages. Patients who engage in limited problem solving restrict their attention to short, repetitive messages with low information content.

THE CONSUMER DECISION PROCESS

Numerous decision-making models have been proposed by marketers over the years. One widely accepted model, shown in Figure 11-2, has three major stages.[9] Prepurchase is the stage in which consumers recognize a need and identify choices to meet that need; it consists of need recognition, information search, and alternative evaluation. Consumption is the actual selection and purchase of a product. Postpurchase describes the evaluation phase of consumer decision-making.

This model can be used to describe decisions ranging from the simple (e.g., habitual and impulse buying) to the complex (e.g., deciding between surgery and drug therapy). Consumers may not consciously go through each step in the model. People who make impulse purchases frequently forgo the prepurchase and postpurchase stages.

Figure 11-2 Stages of consumer decision-making

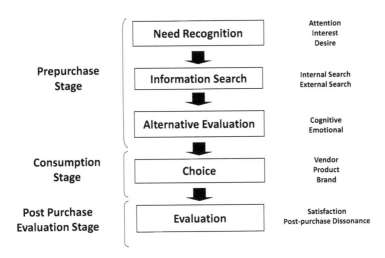

PREPURCHASE

Need Recognition

Consumer decision-making begins with the recognition of a need. This occurs when some stimulus arouses a desire (e.g., a headache arouses a desire to get rid of the pain). Desire-arousing stimuli can be commercial, social, or physical.[9] Commercial stimuli include those commonly associated with the marketing mix, such as a television advertisement or a recommendation from a salesperson. Social stimuli might be a desire to emulate one's peers or word-of-mouth recommendations of friends or family members. Physical stimuli are things such as pain, hunger, and thirst.

Marketers attempt to influence consumer need recognition in numerous ways. They develop promotional messages to directly stimulate the recognition of a need. An advertisement might pose a provocative question ("Are you getting the service you deserve?") or announce new services ("Bone mineral density testing now available").

Marketers also attempt to indirectly induce need recognition by simulating social situations in advertising. Direct-to-consumer drug advertisements often portray attractive people engaged in activities related to drug consumption. An advertisement for an arthritis medication might show an older person playing tennis—the message being that the drug can help you be more active, like this person. A pharmacy advertisement might portray a patient using a computer to access Internet pharmacy services—the message being that it is easy and convenient.

Another way to indirectly induce need recognition is to use sounds, smells, and images to activate physical reactions that lead to consumer purchases. Anyone who has smelled freshly baked bread in a bakery or brewed coffee in a café recognizes the desire that can be stimulated by smells. Music is often piped into stores to affect moods and make consumers more likely to buy. The marketing term *servicescapes* describes the role of facility design features such as lighting, temperature, sound, and signs in influencing consumer behavior.[10]

Despite the best efforts of marketers, however, most stimuli are ineffective in causing need recognition. That is because most are not even noticed. Humans ignore most stimuli, because we are constantly bombarded by commercial messages, social demands, and physical aches and pains. Ignoring them is the only way to survive in this message-laden world. Because people are selective in their attention to stimuli, marketers continually look for innovative ways to break through all of the environmental noise.

The problem with capturing the attention of consumers is exponentially harder in the presence of smart phones and other mobile technology. For instance, the boring wait at the checkout counter used to be a place where retailers could capture the attention of customers to sell magazines and other impulse-purchase items. Today, the customer wait is typically filled with smart phone tasks like checking e-mails, texting, and mobile gaming which can reduce the effectiveness of many point-of-purchase displays and promotional communications at the checkout counter.

To complicate matters for marketers, stimuli that arouse attention do not always arouse sufficient desire to cause action. A smoker may notice and be interested in an advertisement for a smoking cessation program, but the ad may not be sufficient to get the smoker to take action (i.e., enroll in the program). Smokers are continually exposed to commercial, social, and physical messages telling them to quit, but they fail to do so for many reasons, including the perception that the effort it would take to quit is too great.

Information Search

Once a need is recognized, a consumer searches for information about actions that might satisfy the perceived need or want.[11] This can be a simple search of one's memory (called an *internal search*), in which previous experiences or promotional messages are recalled. For instance, a patient who wants information about a nonprescription medication might search her memory for experience with particular brands or information relayed through a television advertisement.

In many cases, the internal memory search is followed by an *external search* for information.[12, 13] In the nonprescription medication example, a consumer might consult a friend, an issue of Consumer Reports magazine, the Internet, or a pharmacist. The level of consumer search depends on several factors:

Whether the decision is a new or repeat one. People who are unfamiliar with the available choices of products or services are more likely to engage in an external search. These people may be more attentive to promotional messages, ask others for recommendations, or engage in research in consumer publications or on the Internet.

Whether products and services are perceived to be different. There is little need for a search when a choice will result in essentially the same outcome. A patient who perceives all pharmacies and pharmacists to be the same will see little reason to engage in an extensive search for a pharmacy. The search may involve simply recalling where the nearest pharmacy is located.

Individual situations and characteristics. Individuals who lack the time, patience, or ability to evaluate information are less likely to engage in a search. Busy people are less likely to spend time choosing nonprescription medications in a community pharmacy. Personal knowledge also influences the level of the search. Individuals with less knowledge of health care are more likely to rely on the opinions of others than to engage in their own search for information.

Several strategies can be used to influence the information search. One is to establish your product or service firmly in the minds of consumers through advertising and other promotional communication. When this has been accomplished, your product or service should be one of the options considered in the consumer's internal memory search. Another strategy is to guide consumers through the external search process with questions and statements such as the following:

- Did your pharmacist check for interactions?
- Not all medicines are alike. Have you ever considered drug y?
- If you have never used drug x, here is what you need to know.
- Are you completely happy with drug x? If not, try drug y.
- Do you ever worry that you are paying too much for drug x?

Evaluation of Alternatives

Once sufficient information has been collected, the consumer can evaluate alternatives. The evaluation can be *cognitive* (thoughtful), or it can be *noncognitive* (emotional). Cognitive evaluation of alternatives involves contemplation and thought. Most consumer behavior models assume a cognitive process. Noncognitive evaluation is less thoughtful, involving intuition or gut feelings.

Noncognitive decisions about care have a greater impact than health professionals may realize. Patients typically choose drugs and health care providers on the basis of feelings, not thoughts. If we have a headache, we don't select a remedy by objective cost–benefit analysis; we simply choose a drug to stop the pain so we can continue what we were doing before the headache began. Our choice of a pharmacist is likely to be determined less by her technical capability than by our feelings when she reassures us about our condition, conveys that she cares about us as people, and helps us feel in control of our health. Even an objective attribute such as low cost may appeal to us more because we feel we are getting a good deal than because of the actual impact on our budget. Many times, our preferences concerning the appearance and features of products and services are based on feelings rather than thoughtful analysis of the pros and cons.

In any evaluation of alternatives, the first step is to identify the important criteria or attributes, such as price and quality of services. This can be difficult for consumers with little knowledge of or experience with the available alternatives. Free trials of products or services provide consumers with some experience. As an added benefit, free trials may encourage consumers to share their experiences with others.

Decisions between alternatives often are based on more than one attribute; this is called multiattribute decision-making. Table 11-1 illustrates a consumer's use of the attributes price, location, and pharmacist relationship to choose a pharmacy. This consumer has chosen to consider only three attributes, possibly because of time limitations or unwillingness to invest more effort in the decision.

Table 11-1 Consumer Assessment of Community Pharmacies

Attribute	Pharmacy A	Pharmacy B	Pharmacy C
Price	Highest in town but still competitive	Competitive	Lowest in town
Location	Near home	Near home and work	Across town
Pharmacist relationship	Excellent and long lasting	No relationship	No relationship

After choosing which attributes to consider, the consumer weighs the relative importance of each and examines how the attributes differ among alternatives (i.e., the competing pharmacies). Some attributes are more important or salient in decision-making than others. Price may be more salient to some consumers, while location or pharmacist relationship may be more salient to others. Clear differences between salient attributes can influence the selection of one alternative over another.

On the other hand, important attributes may have little effect on the final choice. For instance, low drug prices might be expected to be salient in the selection of a pharmacy, but price may be irrelevant to the final choice if the consumer perceives no price difference between competitors.

The attributes that are perceived to differ enough between the alternatives to influence the final choice are called *determinant attributes*. Determinant attributes are those salient attributes that make a difference in choice. For example, highly salient attributes like price and convenient may be perceive a similar between competing pharmacies. Therefore, choice of a pharmacy may be determined by seemingly less important attributes like neatness or general store lighting. Successful pharmacists recognize the importance of paying attention to even minor details when it comes to service, because those details can make the final difference in patient patronage and loyalty.

In Table 11-1, Pharmacy A is the most expensive, but it is near home and the patient has a good relationship with the pharmacist. Pharmacy B has competitive prices and is near work and home, but the patient has no relationship with the pharmacist. Pharmacy C has the lowest prices, but it is across town and again there is no pharmacist relationship. Pharmacy patronage will depend on individual preference.

The reasons for patients' choice of a pharmacy have been studied extensively over the years.[14-19] The research has identified many attributes as salient: convenient location, the pharmacist, patient out-of-pocket cost, convenient hours, friendliness of employees, personalized attention, and specialized services. Attributes that are beyond the control of most pharmacists, such as convenience (i.e., location, operating hours) and out-of-pocket costs to patients, may be determinant. However, pharmacists have the power to influence attributes such as friendliness, personalized attention, professional services, and reliability of care. The extent to which these attributes can determine pharmacy patronage depends on patients, situational factors, and the attributes of competing pharmacies.

CONSUMPTION STAGE

Choice

The prepurchase stage, as described above, prepares consumers for the next stage: making a choice. In truth, consumer choice may consist of several choices. Choosing a nonprescription drug involves choosing a vendor (e.g., drugstore, grocery, mass merchandiser), a channel of distribution (e.g., drive-through, mail order, or Internet pharmacy), and a brand (e.g., generic, store brand, manufacturer brand).

The consumption stage extends beyond product selection and purchase. It also includes the use and disposal of the product which is becoming increasingly important in pharmacy practice.[20-23] The consumption process for a prescription medication encompasses all consumer actions related to the purchase, use, and disposal of the drug. These include selecting a pharmacy, filling and paying for the prescription, taking the medication, and throwing away any medication that has not been consumed.

Decision Rules

Once consumers have determined which criteria to use in making a decision, they make overall judgments based on the criteria and compare them across alternatives. Typically, these judgments follow personal decision rules that the consumer develops through experience.[24]

One consumer decision rule is to apply cutoffs[9]—strict limits for deciding which choices are acceptable and unacceptable. Setting a defined price range (e.g., no more than $10) is a common cutoff rule used by consumers. Prices that fall outside the established range are judged unacceptable.

The application of absolute cutoff rules to decisions is called *noncompensatory decision-making*. Noncompensatory means that deficiencies in some attributes cannot be compensated for by strengths in others. Hence, a product or service with an unacceptable price will not be considered, no matter how favorable the other attributes may be.

Cutoffs can be applied to pharmacy selection. Limits might be established for the distance to a pharmacy, the behavior of pharmacy personnel, and the range of products offered. The use of cutoffs can simplify the decision-making process, but often consumers are left with multiple alternatives that have passed the cutoff rule. Additional decision rules must be used to choose among the remaining alternatives.

Another decision rule used by consumers is to sum the value of the attributes into an overall value for each option. The option with the greatest overall value (i.e., utility) is chosen. Marketers call choices based on overall utility *compensatory decisions*.[9] In compensatory decision-making, the weaknesses of one attribute can be overcome by the strength of another. Thus, consumers may be willing to accept high prices for pharmaceutical services if the quality of those services is perceived to result in significant value.

POSTPURCHASE EVALUATION

Once consumption is completed, consumers evaluate the decision-making process. They evaluate the degree to which their needs and wants have been met, as well as their overall satisfaction with the experience. What was received is compared with what was expected.

During this stage, consumers often have doubts about their choices. They experience cognitive dissonance, particularly when a bad choice could have serious consequences, such as placing personal or financial health at significant risk. Cognitive dissonance is common after people buy an expensive car or a house. They may worry about whether they can afford the purchase and what would happen if something went wrong with what they have bought.

Cognitive dissonance can occur after making health care decisions. Patients may worry about the expense or potential adverse effects associated with a choice. Pharmacists can minimize patients' cognitive dissonance in several ways. One is to make telephone calls to patients a day or two after filling a prescription. This gives the patient an opportunity to communicate concerns to the pharmacist and seek reassurance. Another is to include a notice in the prescription package that encourages the patient to call the pharmacy with questions or visit a Web site for answers to commonly asked questions. Some pharmacies even make money-back guarantees to patients.

"The aim of marketing is to know and
understand the customer so well the product
or service fits him and sells itself."

- Peter Drucker

CUSTOMER JOURNEY

The consumer decision-making model in Figure 11-2 can be used by pharmacists to influence consumer decisions. This helps when designing new services and communicating with customers. Understanding each step in the decision process helps pharmacists offer customer-centered solutions to their needs.

The major concern with the model in Figure 11-2 is that it presents consumer decisions as a linear process where consumers start at one end (need identification) and advance through the model to the end (post-purchase evaluation). Consumer decisions, however, are an iterative process where individuals cycle back and forth through various stages of the decision meanwhile engaging in two-way conversations with the marketer.

Marketers are starting to view the consumer decision process as a circular journey with four stages.[25, 26]

1. Initial Consideration Set: Initial consideration of options after a need is triggered by stimuli which may be physical (pain), social (conversation with a friend), commercial (advertisement), or other type,
2. Active Evaluation: Active addition and subtraction of options through information search (internet search) or shopping (point-of-purchase displays),
3. Moment of Purchase: Selection and completion of the purchase, and
4. Postpurchase: Evaluating the purchase experience and outcome and developing expectations of future purchases.

Although the four-stage customer journey contains many of the same touchpoints as the five-stage consumer decision process, the customer journey sees consumption as a non-linear experience where the consumer is in charge of decisions.

The customer journey has been used as the foundation of several medication use innovations. It was employed to design PillPack, a pharmacy that ships medications to patients in pre-sorted and packaged individualized packets based on the time taken during the day.[27] The customer journey process was also used to elicit an understanding of the factors influencing seasonal flu and tetanus vaccination decisions[28] and smoking cessation.[29] Finally, the customer journey for medication therapy management services was mapped using a process called "Design Thinking."[30] Mapping these journeys lead to insights that were utilized to better serve patients.

In clinical settings, the customer journey becomes the "Patient Journey." The patient journey describes how patients experience a chronic disease or health condition from first becoming aware of the problem through "all stages of presentation, diagnosis, referral and treatment, fulfillment, monitoring, adherence, and follow ups."[31] Understanding each step helps pharmacists identify solutions to overcome the difficult problems and hurdles faced not just by patients, but also the providers seeking to serve those patients. It is applicable to addressing problems of patient nonadherence, medication reconciliation, inpatient and outpatient services, interprofessional care, and almost any complex pharmacist-related process.

VARIABLES AFFECTING CONSUMER DECISION-MAKING

Perception of Risk

Decisions are influenced by the consumer's tolerance for risk. A risk taker is likely to act differently than a risk avoider. Decisions can also be influenced by different types of perceived risk. Perceived risk can be made up of five different types.

1. *Financial risk* refers to financial losses that might occur as a result of a bad purchase, such as overpaying for a nonprescription drug or finding out that a prescription drug is not covered by insurance.
2. *Performance risk* is the possibility that a purchase will not achieve the intended outcome such as when an allergy drug does not relieve allergic symptoms.
3. *Physical risk* is the potential for injury resulting from consumption. For drugs, this might refer to adverse effects or drug interactions.
4. *Social risk* refers to loss of personal social status associated with a purchase. Some drugs, such as those used to treat urinary incontinence or AIDS, can carry a negative social stigma.
5. *Psychological* risk refers to the impact of a purchase on a person's self-esteem. Some drugs have potentially embarrassing adverse effects, such as impotence or flatulence, which can negatively affect self-esteem.

Like most health care decisions, medication use is perceived to be riskier than the average consumer purchase. Those perceptions of risk exist along two dimensions: severity and chance. Severity refers to the significance of a negative impact associated with a decision. With decisions about medications, potential consequences can range in severity from none to pain, suffering, and even death. The greater the perceived severity of a potential outcome, the greater is the risk associated with the decision. Chance refers to the probability of a certain outcome occurring. For drugs, uncertainty about effectiveness, adverse effects, and drug interactions increases perceptions of risk.

Evaluating the risk involved in using pharmacy products and pharmacist services is difficult for most consumers. They lack both the expertise to decide which medications will help their conditions and information on how to use them appropriately. Even after taking a medication, consumers may not know whether it is working unless they receive feedback from the health care provider. Patients need providers to tell them if their cholesterol levels or liver enzymes are too high.

MARKETING IN ACTION

Social risk sometimes trumps physical risk

Sometimes the risk of embarrassment is more important to young people than the risk of sexually transmitted diseases and unintended pregnancy. Despite the well known risks of not using condoms, a study reports that many young people are too embarrassed to buy condoms.[32]

When asked for reasons why they did not buy condoms, students gave a variety of reasons. One commonly reported reason was personal embarrassment leading students to employ various strategies to manage their awkwardness. One out of five young people sought out a clerk of the same sex when purchasing condoms. Another strategy was to conceal the box or buy additional items to distract attention of the clerk at checkout. Some students would postpone condom purchases until no other customers were at the register. Others brought friends along as allies or lied about the reason for purchase, "so the clerk wouldn't get the 'wrong idea.'"

The least embarrassed students reported that buying condoms was "the responsible thing to do." Study authors concluded that if the idea of social responsibility is stressed to students, condom purchases may increase.

Source: Reference[32]

Involvement

Involvement is defined as the consumer's perception of the importance of a person, object, or situation.[9] It describes an internal state of arousal, preparedness, and attention. Involvement is an indicator of motivation because it signals personal relevance. Sick people pay more attention to health messages than healthy people do, because the messages are more relevant to their personal situation. The degree of consumer involvement can vary from moment to moment, depending on a person's changing situation.

Involvement is an important concept for pharmacists, because consumers who are interested in their health and health care behave differently than those who are not.[33-36] Involvement is positively related to extended problem solving. Interested consumers are more alert to health information, committed to their therapeutic plan, and likely to work with professionals to achieve good therapeutic outcomes. In addition, involvement is important because it influences consumer decision-making.

The information search, information processing, and susceptibility to persuasion are affected by the consumer's involvement.[9] Involved consumers spend more time and effort searching for information that relates to purchase and consumption. They are more thoughtful in their actions, understand information better, and have greater ability to recall details later. Also, involved people are more likely to listen to persuasive arguments.

Involvement is necessary for thoughtful behavior, which is needed when dealing with important, complex decisions such as those about health care. Participation in health care decision-making requires consumers to fully understand their choices and the consequences. This means consumers should be attentive to information and thoughtful in their choices. Consumers who are not thoughtful are more likely to make decisions on the basis of emotions, habit, or random choice. Involvement with pharmaceuticals and pharmacy services is influenced by several factors:[9]

- o Personal relevance of the object to the consumer. Although pharmacists may perceive their services as critically important, patients may not consider these services crucial. The relevance of anything is determined by the perspective of the individual.

- o The product or service being considered. Some things are inherently more important to people than others. Health care is considered a high-involvement activity in comparison with the purchase of commodities such as laundry detergent. Involvement with health care is related to the perceived risk associated with its purchase and consumption and the potential benefit it can provide to meet personal needs. The more that people realize the potential benefit or risk associated with specific health care decisions, the greater their attention and involvement.

- o The situation. Many healthy people ignore health care issues—until they get sick. Then they become actively involved in finding a way to treat their illness. Their involvement is situation dependent. When the illness is resolved, the need for involvement changes, and the person often falls back into his or her previous low level of involvement.

Customizing Services to Patient Involvement

Pharmacists who understand their patients' level of involvement can use that knowledge to tailor educational and counseling information and stimulate greater involvement.[37] Standardized surveys are available for measuring involvement, but they are rarely necessary. Most pharmacists can assess a patient's involvement level by observing body language, eye contact, and responses to questions about treatments.

Patients who are highly involved can receive more complex messages and greater amounts of information. These patients will be receptive and pay attention. Persuasive messages are also more effective with involved patients, because they are more willing to follow the logic and information associated with persuasive arguments.

For low-involvement patients, relatively simple, short, repetitive messages are better. A smaller amount of information should be provided in plain language. Repetition of crucial messages helps low-involvement patients to retain information long enough to influence behavior.

Enhancing Patient Involvement

Pharmacists can enhance their patients' involvement and help make them more receptive to the complex health messages that are commonly part of the practice of pharmaceutical care. Greater involvement can be stimulated in the following ways:[37]

- Expertise can be increased by educating patients about their diseases and medication therapy. Pharmacists can convey to patients the role of pharmacy services in achieving positive health outcomes.

- Opportunity to process information can be enhanced by reducing the number of distractions and providing a quiet counseling area for conversations with patients. Opportunity can also be increased by scheduling patient counseling sessions at hours convenient for both the pharmacist and the patient.

- When patients have limited expertise and opportunity, pharmacists should adjust counseling strategies to the patient's level. Pharmacists should provide only as much information as the patient can adequately process and should simplify the message for patients with less education or reduced cognitive ability.

Pharmacists need to understand consumer involvement, because it affects the way information is processed. Effective medication counseling requires that the patient receive and understand the message being conveyed by the pharmacist. Insufficient mental involvement of the patient in the counseling transaction can lead to misunderstanding and ultimate therapeutic failure.

Engagement

Engagement is related, but distinctly different from involvement. Engagement is the capability and participation of customers in the co-production or use of a product or service. Originally discussed in reference to participation in social media,[38] it described the various levels of participation in media ranging from passive observation of the media postings of other people to creation and posting of original content for the use of others.

In health care, patient engagement refers to a patient's willingness and ability to manage his or her own health and care plus active participation in care.[39] Evidence indicates that patients who are actively engaged in their health care have better health outcomes and often lower costs.[39-41] Consequently, health care organizations are trying to increase patient engagement through education, rewards, and collaborative decision making.

An element of patient engagement is *patient activation* which refers to a patient's ability and willingness to manage his or her own health and care.[39] It is measured with a standardized instrument called the *patient activation measure* (PAM).[42]

According to PAM, patient activation has four levels. Level 1, patients are starting to take a role in their therapy but are still passive because they lack confidence in their capabilities. Level 2, patients begin to develop knowledge and confidence and take the beginning steps toward engagement. Level 3, individuals take concrete action to engage, while in Level 4, individuals work at maintaining their newly adopted engagement in their care. Much still needs to be learned about patient activation. It has been associated with patient medication adherence and improved outcomes,[43] but it shows promise as a tool to improve patient outcomes.

MARKETING IN ACTION

Sharing Medications

A literature review found that sharing prescription medications is common.[44] The prevalence of borrowing ranged from 5% to 50% depending on the population studied, and lending prescription medications to others was done by 6% to 23% of people. Medicines were shared between family members, friends, and acquaintances. Some drugs were more commonly shared than others.

One US study found that adults were more likely to share allergy medications, pain medications, and antibiotics. Acne medications have also been found to be widely shared. Another study indicated that birth control medications are commonly shared. Dermatology patients frequently shared prescription topical corticosteroids and other dermatologic medications. Alarmingly, some studies even showed patients sharing antidiabetic, cardiovascular, and antihypertensive medications.

When asked to explain reasons for sharing, patients reported that the main reason was running out of their medicine and knowing someone with the same medical problem who was willing to share. Other reasons for borrowing were related to affordability, if the situation was an emergency, or for convenience. Lending of leftover medications was common.

The complexity of the problem suggests that multiple interventions may be needed to reduce borrowing and lending of medications. One solution is to encourage parents to model good medication taking practices for their children. Another is to educate people about the risks of sharing medications. Making medications more affordable and offering programs that remind patients to get their prescriptions filled are other solutions.

Perception of Control

Control refers to consumers' perceptions that they can influence their personal situations and environment. Control is a fundamental desire of humans, and low levels of control are associated with high levels of stress. In pharmacists, lack of control is associated with job burnout.[45]

It is important for consumers to feel that they control the pharmacy service experience. Consumers who sense that they lack control are more likely to become dissatisfied and act to regain control. Consumers who see a long check-out line in a pharmacy may exert control by attempting to find another check-out line, continue shopping until the line becomes shorter, or leave the pharmacy without making a purchase.

Marketers use several strategies to increase a consumer's feeling of control. One is to provide detailed feedback about the consumer's progress in the service sequence. This helps the consumer know what will happen next and how long it will take to complete the process. Feedback about the service process helps consumers reset overoptimistic expectations and gives them information to make an informed choice about whether to wait. Then, a 30 minute wait to fill a prescription becomes a conscious choice rather than something that is inflicted upon them.

Another strategy is to increase choice. Consumers who can select among various options feel more in control. However, too many options can make consumers feel overwhelmed and frustrated. Two or three alternatives are usually sufficient.

Finally, marketers often try to make service experiences as consistent and predictable as possible. At most chain pharmacies or mass merchandisers, consumers find little variation among stores. That is because consumers like to know that the CVS or Walgreens in a distant town will be similar to the one in their neighborhood. The ability to find merchandise and services at any store gives consumers the perception of control over their purchase and the service experience.

INTEGRATING MODELS

Table 11-2 shows how consumer behavior variables relate to the consumer decision process. Perceptions of risk are more likely to influence the later stages of the process while involvement affects the beginning stages. Engagement should influence all stages of consumer decision making. Control should influence the search, evaluation, and choice of alternatives.

Table 11-2 How consumer behavior variables affect the consumer decision process

	Before			During	After
	Need Recognition	Information Search	Evaluation of Alternatives	Choice	Post-Purchase Evaluation
Perception of Risk		X	X	X	X
Involvement	X	X	X		
Engagement	X	X	X	X	X
Perceptions of Control		X	X	X	

HEALTH BEHAVIOR MODELS

In addition to the models of consumer behavior discussed in the preceding sections, other models can help pharmacists understand health behaviors. The three most commonly cited in the pharmacy literature are listed in Table 11-3. Any clinical intervention by pharmacists should consult these or other health behavior models to develop an evidence-based approach to care. Otherwise, pharmacists are likely to make avoidable errors in treating patients. For a detailed description of these models and other models, consult Theory at a Glance: A Guide for Health Promotion Practice.[46]

Table 11-3 Common Health Behavior Models Used in Pharmacy Practice

Theory	Description	Pharmacy Practice Examples
Health Belief Model	A consumer's likelihood of taking action to prevent or treat a health condition is determined by his or her perception of susceptibility to that condition, the severity of the condition, the benefits of taking action, the costs of taking action, and the barriers to taking action.	Osteoporosis screening[47], use of herpes zoster vaccinations,[48] impact of cost sharing,[49] and warfarin adherence[50]
Theory of Reasoned Action/Theory of Planned Behavior	A person's intentions to act (quit smoking) predict actual behavior. Changing behavior starts with influencing beliefs, attitudes, perceptions, and intentions about a behavior through education, counseling, support services, and persuasive messages.	Pharmacist intention to provide MTM,[51]non-prescription medicines,[52] substance abuse,[53] and collaboration between pharmacists and physicians[54]
Transtheoretical Model	People progress through five stages of readiness to change their health behaviors; precontemplation, contemplation, preparation, action, and maintenance. The success of behavior-change strategies depends on what stage the person is in.	Smoking cessation,[55] pharmacist counseling,[56] and treatment discontinuation[57]

SUMMARY

Understanding the behavior of consumers is an essential part of marketing pharmacy products and pharmacist services. Pharmacists can benefit from understanding some basic principles of consumer behavior. They can use this knowledge to influence patient medication compliance, change smoking behavior, advertise services, design services, and influence physician prescribing.

Reference List

(1) Tversky A, Kahneman D. The framing of decisions and the psychology of choice. Science 1981;211(4481):453-458.

(2) Tversky A, Kahneman D. Judgment under Uncertainty: Heuristics and Biases. Science 1974;185(4157):1124-1131.

(3) Himmelstein DU, Ariely D, Woolhandler S. Pay-for-performance: toxic to quality? Insights from behavioral economics. Int J Health Serv 2014;44(2):203-214.

(4) Waber RL, Shiv B, Carmon Z, Ariely D. Commercial features of placebo and therapeutic efficacy. JAMA 2008;299(9):1016-1017.

(5) Christakis NA, Fowler JH. The Collective Dynamics of Smoking in a Large Social Network. N Engl J Med 2008;358(21):2249-2258.

(6) Christakis NA, Fowler JH. The Spread of Obesity in a Large Social Network over 32 Years. N Engl J Med 2007;357(4):370-379.

(7) Rosenquist JN, Murabito J, Fowler JH, Christakis NA. The Spread of Alcohol Consumption Behavior in a Large Social Network. Annals of Internal Medicine 2010;152(7):426-433.

(8) Physician Office Visitors Are 'Drug Store Super Shoppers'. Drug Store News . 11-17-2014.

(9) Engel JF, Blackwell RD, Miniard PW. Consumer Behavior. Fort Worth, TX: Dryden Press; 1993.

(10) Lin BY, Leu WJ, Breen GM, Lin WH. Servicescape: physical environment of hospital pharmacies and hospital pharmacists' work outcomes. Health Care Manage Rev 2008;33(2):156-168.

(11) DeLorme DE, Huh J, Reid LN. Source Selection in Prescription Drug Information Seeking and Influencing Factors: Applying the Comprehensive Model of Information Seeking in an American Context. Journal of Health Communication 2011;16(7):766-787.

(12) Kim WJ, King KW. Product Category Effects on External Search for Prescription and Nonprescription Drugs. Journal of Advertising 2009;38(1):5-20.

(13) Delonia OC, Vivek M. How did you find your physician? Intl J of Pharm & Health Mrkt 2009;3(1):46-58.

(14) Patterson BJ, Doucette WR, Urmie JM, McDonough RP. Exploring relationships among pharmacy service use, patronage motives, and patient satisfaction. J Am Pharm Assoc (2003) 2013;53(4):382-389.

(15) Franic DM, Haddock SM, Tucker LT, Wooten N. Pharmacy patronage: identifying key factors in the decision making process using the determinant attribute approach. J Am Pharm Assoc (2003) 2008;48(1):71-85.

(16) Shannon GW, Cromley EK, Fink JL, III. Pharmacy patronage among the elderly: selected racial and geographical patterns. Soc Sci Med 1985;20(1):85-93.

(17) Baldwin HJ, Riley DA, Wojcik AF. Prescription purchasers' patronage motives. Pharm Manage Comb Am J Pharm 1979;151(4):185-190.

(18) Gagnon JP. Factors affecting pharmacy patronage motives-a literature review. Journal of American Pharmaceutical Association 1977;556--59, 566.

(19) Herman CM, Wills RA, Jr. A demographic analysis--community pharmacy patronage. J Am Pharm Assoc 1974;14(2):66-70.

(20) Perry LA, Shinn BW, Stanovich J. Quantification of an ongoing community-based medication take-back program. J Am Pharm Assoc (2003) 2014;54(3):275-279.

(21) James TH, Helms ML, Braund R. Analysis of medications returned to community pharmacies. Ann Pharmacother 2009;43(10):1631-1635.

(22) Stewart H, Malinowski A, Ochs L, Jaramillo J, McCall K, III, Sullivan M. Inside Maine's Medicine Cabinet: Findings From the Drug Enforcement Administration's Medication Take-Back Events. Am J Public Health 2015;105(1):e65-e71.

(23) Judith AS, Lisa MN, Nick B, Malcolm M. The global public health issue of pharmaceutical waste: what role for pharmacists? JGR 2014;5(1):126-137.

(24) Riva S, Monti M, Antonietti A. Simple heuristics in over-the-counter drug choices: a new hint for medical education and practice. Adv Med Educ Pract 2011;2:59-70.

(25) Court D, Elzinga D, Mulder S, Vetvik OJ. The consumer journey. McKinsey Quarterly [June]. 2009.

(26) David WN, Pine II BJ. Using the customer journey to road test and refine the business model. Strategy & Leadership 2013;41(2):12-17.

(27) Parker TJ. Prescribing Design. Design Management Review 2014;25(3):30-33.

(28) Wheelock A, Miraldo M, Parand A, Vincent C, Sevdalis N. Journey to vaccination: a protocol for a multinational qualitative study. BMJ Open 2014;4(1).

(29) Kimbell L. Designing for Service as One Way of Designing Services. International Journal of Design 2011;5(2).

(30) Isetts BJ, Schommer JC, Westberg SM, Johnson JK, Froiland NHJM. Evaluation of a Consumer-Generated Marketing Plan for Medication Therapy Management Services . Innovations in Pharmacy 2012;3(1).

(31) Gupta M, von Allmen H, Seiter S, Jaffe H. A new foundation for designing winning brand strategies: The Patient Journey re-envisioned. New York,NY: IMS Consulting Group; 2014.

(32) Nagourney E. Behavior: Sweaty Palms at the Pharmacy. New York Times 2004 Dec 24.

(33) Sansgiry SS, Cady PS, Sansgiry S. Consumer Involvement. Health Marketing Quarterly 2001;19(1):61-78.

(34) Sansgiry SS, Cady PS, Sansgiry S. Consumer involvement: effects on information processing from over-the-counter medication labels. Health Mark Q 2001;19(1):61-78.

(35) Gore P, Madhavan S, McClung G, Riley D. Consumer involvement in nonprescription medicine purchase decisions. J Health Care Mark 1994;14(2):16-23.

(36) Lipowski EE. How consumers choose a pharmacy. Am Pharm 1993;NS33(12 Suppl):S14-S17.

(37) Holdford D, Watrous M. Relative importance consumers place on pharmaceutical services. Journal of Pharmaceutical Marketing Management 11[4], 55-68. 1997.

(38) Hollebeek LD, Glynn MS, Brodie RJ. Consumer Brand Engagement in Social Media: Conceptualization, Scale Development and Validation. Journal of Interactive Marketing 2014;28(2):149-165.

(39) James J. Health Policy Brief: Patient Activation. Health Aff (Millwood) 2013.

(40) Hibbard JH, Greene J. What The Evidence Shows About Patient Activation: Better Health Outcomes And Care Experiences; Fewer Data On Costs. Health Affairs 2013;32(2):207-214.

(41) Greene J, Hibbard JH. Why does patient activation matter? An examination of the relationships between patient activation and health-related outcomes. J Gen Intern Med 2012;27(5):520-526.

(42) Hibbard JH, Stockard J, Mahoney ER, Tusler M. Development of the Patient Activation Measure (PAM): Conceptualizing and Measuring Activation in Patients and Consumers. Health Services Research 2004;39(4):1005-1026.

(43) Parchman ML, Zeber JE, Palmer RF. Participatory decision making, patient activation, medication adherence, and intermediate clinical outcomes in type 2 diabetes: a STARNet study. Ann Fam Med 2010;8(5):410-417.

(44) Beyene KA, Sheridan J, Aspden T. Prescription medication sharing: a systematic review of the literature. Am J Public Health 2014;104(4):e15-e26.

(45) Lahoz MR, Mason HL. Burnout among pharmacists. Am Pharm 1990;NS30(8):28-32.

(46) National Cancer Institute. Theory at a Glance: A Guide for Health Promotion Practice . 2nd ed. 2005.

(47) Deo P, Nayak R, Rajpura J. Women's Attitudes and Health Beliefs toward Osteoporosis Screening in a Community Pharmacy. J Osteoporos 2013;2013:650136.

(48) Hurley LP, Lindley MC, Harpaz R et al. Barriers to the use of herpes zoster vaccine. Ann Intern Med 2010;152(9):555-560.

(49) Zeber JE, Grazier KL, Valenstein M, Blow FC, Lantz PM. Effect of a medication copayment increase in veterans with schizophrenia. Am J Manag Care 2007;13(6 Pt 2):335-346.

(50) Orensky IA, Holdford DA. Predictors of noncompliance with warfarin therapy in an outpatient anticoagulation clinic. Pharmacotherapy 2005;25(12):1801-1808.

(51) Herbert KE, Urmie JM, Newland BA, Farris KB. Prediction of pharmacist intention to provide Medicare medication therapy management services using the theory of planned behavior. Res Social Adm Pharm 2006;2(3):299-314.

(52) Theppanya K, Suwannapong N, Howteerakul N. Health-science students' self-efficacy, social support, and intention to work in rural areas of the Lao People's Democratic Republic. Rural Remote Health 2014;14:2530.

(53) Roberto AJ, Shafer MS, Marmo J. Predicting substance-abuse treatment providers' communication with clients about medication assisted treatment: a test of the theories of reasoned action and planned behavior. J Subst Abuse Treat 2014;47(5):307-313.

(54) Kucukarslan S, Lai S, Dong Y, Al-Bassam N, Kim K. Physician beliefs and attitudes toward collaboration with community pharmacists. Res Social Adm Pharm 2011;7(3):224-232.

(55) Kennedy DT, Small RE. Development and implementation of a smoking cessation clinic in community pharmacy practice. J Am Pharm Assoc (Wash) 2002;42(1):83-92.

(56) Taylor J, Berger B, Anderson-Harper H, Grimley D. Pharmacists' readiness to assess consumers' over-the-counter product selections. J Am Pharm Assoc (Wash) 2000;40(4):487-494.

(57) Berger BA, Hudmon KS, Liang H. Predicting treatment discontinuation among patients with multiple sclerosis: application of the transtheoretical model of change. J Am Pharm Assoc (2003) 2004;44(4):445-454.

Chapter Questions

1. What economic, social, and personal influences affected your decision to become a pharmacist? What influences will determine your career choices?

2. Identify decisions in health care that you consider risky and not risky. How might perceptions of risk affect how patients progress through each stage of the consumer decision-making model in Figure 11-2?

3. Discuss the different types of risk faced by patients who are seeking treatment for migraine headaches.

4. Name several pharmaceutical products. Classify them into what you perceive to be high and low involvement categories. How might you counsel patients differently about high versus low involvement products?

5. In general terms, discuss the value of consumer behavior models. How can a pharmacist use them to better influence patient behavior?

Activities

1. Select a significant purchase you have made and describe both your thoughts and your actions as you proceeded through each of the decision- making steps of (1) need recognition, (2) information search, (3) evaluation of alternatives, (4) consumption, and (5) postpurchase evaluation.

2. Select one of the following health behavior models and describe how pharmacists can use it to help patients take their medications correctly.
>   a. Health belief model.
>   b. Theory of reasoned action/theory of planned behavior.
>   c. Transtheoretical model.

CHAPTER **12**

MARKET SEGMENTATION

Objectives

After studying this chapter, the reader should be able to

- o   Define market segmentation, targeting, and positioning
- o   Discuss the purpose of market segmentation
- o   List characteristics of desirable market segments
- o   Describe ways in which pharmacists can segment their markets, and give examples of each
- o   Suggest several ways in which practicing pharmacists can conduct market research
- o   Discuss the steps involved in segmenting markets

Segmenting customers into groups is a fundamental part of marketing. Marketers realize that it is undesirable to try to serve all potential customers in a market, because each customer has different needs, wants, habits, and circumstances. The only way to satisfy everyone in a market would be to offer an infinite array of products and services at any time or place, free of charge!

Instead, marketers attempt to identify those individuals in the market who can be served most effectively and profitably. This process, called *segmentation*, is accomplished by categorizing individuals in the market according to shared characteristics, such as age, buying habits, or lifestyle. Those characteristics are used as a basis for developing a marketing mix that is targeted to groups' special needs, wants, and behaviors. When pharmacists use customer targeting in their practice, they are simply identifying those individuals they can and want to serve. This chapter explains how pharmacists can use market segmentation to more effectively serve their customers and patients.

When you try to please everyone, you rarely please anyone.

—Anonymous

Marketers use segmentation to identify similarities within groups of consumers and benefit from these similarities. Although every person in the world is different, it is still useful to group people according to consistent characteristics and make generalizations about these groups. Such generalizations can help marketers serve their customers better. Marketers who practice market segmentation are in a better position to:

o *Identify opportunities in the market.* Opportunities exist when not all customer segments are served well. Segmentation helps identify poorly served and profitable segments of the population.

o *Tailor a unique marketing mix.* Segmentation permits the targeting of specific customer groups, to which a unique mix of price, product, promotion, and place can be offered.

o *Charge and receive higher prices.* A unique marketing mix can enhance customers' perceptions of value and allow higher prices to be charged.

o *Serve customers more efficiently.* Segmentation permits an organization to specialize. It can be more efficient to offer specialized services and products for only a few segments instead of maintaining the capacity to serve all customers.

o *Gain a competitive advantage.* Organizations that can identify market opportunities and offer a unique marketing mix can have an advantage over competitors.

In the past, segmentation was less important in the development of marketing strategy. In the mid-20th century, companies were able to meet consumer needs by using a mass marketing strategy—one that attempts to serve the entire market with the same marketing mix, offering every consumer the same price, location, promotion, and product mix. Because there was tremendous demand for products and services at that time, sellers who offered a uniform marketing mix to customers could succeed.

Today, mass marketing is no longer an effective strategy because there is too much competition for consumer demand. Pharmaceuticals now can be purchased at grocery stores, mass merchandisers, independents, chains, franchises, clinics, and physicians' offices. Drug products can be obtained through mail order, telephone, vending machines, drive-through pharmacies, and the Internet. Information about those pharmaceuticals can be found in seconds on the internet or mobile devices.

Marketers that use a mass marketing strategy to meet consumer needs now find it impossible to compete with marketers that practice segmentation. Competitors that use segmentation can lure away the most profitable segments of the mass market with unique promotional appeals, services, product features, and the like. Over time, the mass marketer is left with only the least profitable customers.

SEGMENTATION, TARGETING, AND POSITIONING

The terminology associated with market segmentation can be confusing. Segmentation is often referred to indirectly with terms such as target marketing, niche marketing, target groups, and demographics. When people use these terms, they are usually speaking of segmentation.

Market segmentation can be defined as dividing a market on the basis of differences and forming subgroups based on common characteristics. Individuals in markets can be segmented by sex, age, behavior, and other characteristics. Pharmacists may segment their patients by disease state; this is useful because knowing a person's disease state can help a pharmacist understand the amount and types of services that person might need.

Market segmentation goes hand in hand with *targeting* and *positioning*. Segmentation identifies variables that can be used to target desirable groups of individuals. A pharmacist who wants to serve the osteoporosis market can use sex and age as a basis of segmenting the market. Within the osteoporosis market, women over the age of 65 may be targeted, because they are at increased risk for fractures. On the basis of unique characteristics of this segment, a marketing mix can be chosen that clearly positions pharmacist-directed osteoporosis services in the minds of targeted customers. Pharmacists may attempt to position themselves in the minds of patients as "the drug expert" or "the most accessible health professional." Positioning is achieved through promotional communications, the merchandise and services offered, and other elements of the marketing mix.

IDENTIFYING DESIRABLE MARKET SEGMENTS

Segmentation is useful only if it provides some competitive advantage in serving customers. The challenge is to determine which customer segments are desirable. Desirable market segments need the following characteristics:

- *The segment must be identifiable.* It is easy to identify patients who fall into demographic categories defined by age, sex, and income. Other classifications may be difficult for most pharmacists to use. A segment labeled "hypochondriacs" would not be desirable if individuals in the segment were not easily distinguished from "non-hypochondriacs."

- *The segment must be accessible.* Pharmacists need to be able to reach each market segment with a customized marketing mix. Segments must be accessible both for the delivery of the product and for promotional communications. Using the hypochondriac example above, marketers would need to identify where individuals in the segment could be found, what media they are exposed to, and ways they could be easily reached and served.

- *The segment must be of sufficient size.* Customer segments must be large enough to be profitable to an organization. Since segments often require a customized marketing mix, the segment must have enough revenue-generating potential to cover the extra costs associated with customization. Thus, current and future revenue associated with each segment must be estimated.

- *The segment must be responsive to your targeted marketing mix.* The value of segmentation lies in identifying segments that are more responsive to your targeted marketing mix than to those of your competitors. If a targeted mix cannot satisfy the market segment better than the mix offered to the general market, then segmentation provides little advantage.

SELECTING SEGMENTATION VARIABLES

Segmentation variables are used as surrogates for behavior. Knowing a patient's age and disease state is useful in segmentation because these variables are associated with levels of prescription drug use. Segmentation variables should be chosen on the basis of their relationship to the behavior in which you are interested.

Selecting variables to use in segmenting markets can be relatively simple. Much of the information needed for segmentation already exists in patient databases or in a pharmacist's personal knowledge of customers. Segmentation becomes difficult only as more complex multivariate analyses of the market are conducted. Pharmacists can choose segmentation variables in several ways:

- ○ *Through experience and intuition.* Pharmacists often rely on personal experience and judgment to identify and evaluate customer segments in a market. Most experienced pharmacists have a good idea of the needs, tendencies, and characteristics of their patients.

- ○ *By adopting the ideas of others.* Professional pharmacy organizations (e.g., American Pharmacists Association, American Society of Health-System Pharmacists, National Association of Chain Drug Stores, and National Community Pharmacists Association) and publications such as *Drug Topics, Pharmacy Times,* and *U.S. Pharmacist* present interesting ideas about segmenting the market for pharmacy services and products. Pharmacists can often find ways to apply these ideas to their settings.

- ○ *By analyzing customer data.* Pharmacists can analyze data collected from prescription records, customer databases, and consumer surveys, as well as data purchased from market research companies, to select segmentation variables. The key is to analyze the information in a way that provides unique insight into behaviors of individuals within specific market segments.

EMPIRICAL VERSUS HYPOTHESIS -DRIVEN APPROACHES

A segmentation approach can be empirical or hypothesis driven. In empirical segmentation, the marketer's choice of segmentation variables is based on professional experience or information collected from the literature. This approach resembles empirical treatment by physicians (i.e., making clinical decisions on the basis of professional knowledge). Pharmacists might use empirical segmentation to classify patients by disease state, frequency of drug use, and age—characteristics that have well known associations with the need for medication therapy management.

In hypothesis-driven segmentation, the marketer tests hypotheses about the relationships between market segmentation variables (e.g., demographics, benefits sought) and outcomes (e.g., utilization, sales, and adherence). The purpose is to gain insights about actual and potential customers that can be used to secure a competitive advantage. Hypothesis-driven segmentation builds on information used in empirical segmentation, such as the opinions of managers and published information. However, it goes further by relying on market research techniques to identify patterns of consumer behavior. These techniques can include qualitative research (e.g., focus groups, personal interviews) as well as multivariate research methods (e.g., conjoint analysis, logistic regression, structural equation modeling). Pharmacists with good people skills and common sense may be able to conduct their own focus groups and personal interviews. For multivariate research, pharmacists usually contract with marketing research firms or universities. It is common for researchers at universities and contract research organizations to analyze demographic, drug-use, and insurance plan information to identify variables that help predict drug utilization patterns.

Both empirical and hypothesis-driven segmentation methods have advantages and disadvantages for marketers. Empirical segmentation relies on the marketer's experience and ability to understand which variables are useful. This experience is gained from reading business and professional publications and conducting business every day. It is only as expensive as the amount of time devoted to it and the cost of the subscriptions to publications. It is a time-tested method; business owners have relied on their intuition and knowledge to serve customers for thousands of years.

The problem with empirical segmentation is that life in today's world is so complex. Managers are bombarded daily with tremendous amounts of information about customer behavior and the actions of competitors. Even if they are able to keep up with all of the insights offered in business and professional publications, this may not provide an advantage, since competitors have access to the same information. Managers often find it useful to get help in identifying patterns of behavior that will offer a competitive advantage.

Hypothesis-driven segmentation uses methods from a variety of fields to gain greater understanding of consumer behavior and markets. Marketers borrow from psychology, sociology, anthropology, computer science, economics, communications, and other fields to propose and test hypotheses about markets. The methods can be as rigorous as anything found in medicine or the basic sciences.

In general, the more rigorous the methods used in hypothesis-driven segmentation are, the higher the cost. Thus, larger companies or professional associations are more likely to use this type of research. Nevertheless, smaller firms can conduct simple hypothesis-driven research on current and potential customers. An independent pharmacist could use patient profiles to identify utilization data associated with patients' requests for help with their medications. The pharmacist might hypothesize that greater numbers of medications, changes in therapy, specific disease states, and specific age groups are associated with requests for help. The pharmacist could then test whether these variables can consistently predict requests for help. If so, specific patients who might need greater pharmacist assistance could be targeted.

NICHE MARKETING

A niche is a small, narrowly defined market, so niche marketing focuses on serving narrow subsets of overall markets. Pharmacists who use niche strategies select a single, profitable segment that offers the best opportunity for success. This niche might be a disease state, product line, specialty medicine, or specific patient need. Ideally, marketers should choose niches that are (1) large enough to be profitable, (2) underserved or ignored by competitors, and (3) able to be exploited by the unique skills and capabilities of the marketers.

Figure 12-1 shows how the osteoarthritis market might be segmented by using differentiation, niche, and microniche strategies. Osteoarthritis patients could be grouped into those with mild, moderate, and severe osteoarthritis and according to method of payment: Medicaid, private insurance, and self-pay. A differentiation strategy might target the self-pay and Medicaid markets, with elements in the marketing mix specific to patients in each segment. Although the pharmacist will continue to serve the untargeted private insurance segment, no special effort will be made to meet the needs of this segment.

Alternatively, a more focused, niche strategy might aim to serve only self-pay patients. A microniche strategy might even limit efforts to the mild osteoarthritis, self-pay market.

Figure 12-1 Segmenting the osteoarthritis market using differentiation, niche, and microniche strategies.

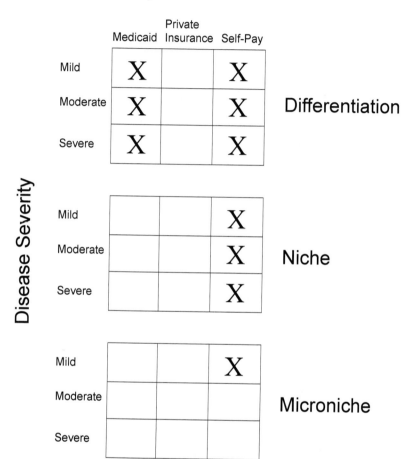

A common assumption is that a business's largest segment should be targeted, but this strategy is not always the most appropriate. The largest patient segment for many pharmacies is made up of patients who want fast and cheap drugs with minimal services. The competition for this segment is often fierce, and its contribution to profits can be slim, especially if third-party insurance reimbursements are low. Pharmacists may find it more profitable and satisfying to target smaller, more lucrative segments such as pediatric patients with chronic diseases or women at risk for osteoporosis.

DEMOGRAPHIC SEGMENTATION

The most common ways of segmenting markets are demographic, geographic, psychographic, behavioral–utilization, and benefits segmentation (Table 12-1). Markets are most easily segmented according to demographic and geographic categories. Demographics are descriptive statistics that quantify populations and subpopulations at specific points in time. Demographic variables such as age, sex, income, and ethnicity can be used to subdivide the market. Demographic data about consumer markets are widely available from numerous public and private sources, many of which can be accessed on the Internet.

Table 12-1 Common Ways of Segmenting Markets

Basis of Segmentation	Segmentation Categories	Examples
Demographic	Age, sex, family size, income, occupation, education, family life cycle, religious affiliation, nationality	Family life cycle: newlywed, married with young children, married with older children, empty nesters
Geographic	Country, region, metropolitan statistical area, city, county, state, neighborhood, rural	Region: Northeast, Midwest, Northwest, Southwest, Southeast
Psychographic	Personality, lifestyle, values	Lifestyles: health hermits, recluses, ailing outgoers, health indulgers
Behavioral	Actual behavior: frequency of use, situations, user status, loyalty, adoption of innovations	Willingness to adopt innovations: innovators, early adopters, early majority, late majority, laggards
	Potential behavior: readiness to buy or act	
	Mixed behavior: variables at risk for drug-related problems	
Benefits	Benefits sought are varied and almost endless	Quality buyers, service buyers, value buyers, economy buyers

The internet has made access to demographic information very easy. Census data available on the Internet at www .census.gov contain demographic information including sex, age, race, Hispanic origin, household type, housing occupancy, homeowners, renters, school enrollment, educational attainment, marital status, disability status, labor force status, commuting, occupation, income and benefits, and poverty. Industry specific information can also be found (NAICS: 44611 - Pharmacies and drug stores). If census data is too general for individual businesses, more detailed demographic data can be purchased from private market research companies and local chambers of commerce.

Demographics constitute one of the most common bases of segmentation, because it is easy to classify people according to age, sex, and other demographic variables. Furthermore, consumer behavior is often linked to demographics. For instance, women use health care services and prescription drugs more frequently than men do.[1] Women also know more about health matters, are more likely to seek health information, and more frequently use preventive care and nonprescription medications.[2]

Demographics are useful in developing targeting strategies. Knowing the age and makeup of households (e.g., sex, marital status, number of children) can help pharmacists target key decision makers in the selection and administration of prescription drugs. Data on the average income in a neighborhood can indicate consumers' available resources. Information about the percentage of full-time workers in an area can give insight into the amount of time customers have available for shopping and health care.

MARKETING IN ACTION

Segmenting Females

Globally, women control trillions of dollars in annual consumer spending When summed, the market for women is twice as big as the markets of China and India combined.[3] Pharmacists should have an effective strategy for marketing to women. One way is to see women not as a single market but a number of submarkets.

1. For example, when gender was linked to other demographic information like education, disposable income, and stage of life, marketers identified six key female consumer segments.[3]

2. *Fast-Tracker*: women who are elite economically and educationally. They seek adventure and learning. Sub-segments consist of Striving *for Achievement* in which job and recognition are priorities and *Independent Women* who work the most and prize personal autonomy.

3. *Pressure Cooker*: women who are married with children and feel ignored and stereotyped. Subsegments are *Successful Multitaskers* who feel in control

and *Struggling for Stability* who feel they are constantly battling the chaos of life.

4.   *Relationship Focused:* are content and optimistic, are not pressed for time, have ample discretionary income, and focus on experiences, not products.

5.   *Managing on Her Own*: are single again, divorced, or widowed who are seeking connections in their lives.

6.   *Fulfilled Empty Nester*: are satisfied and free to pursue their desires. They are concerned about health and aging gracefully focused on travel, exercise, and leisure.

7.   *Making Ends Meet*: have no discretionary money, often lacking a college education, and looking for value and small luxuries.

Source: Reference [3]

The Senior Segment

Health care providers have given much attention to the market for older Americans. The senior market segment is one of the greatest users of prescription medications and other forms of health care. Seniors make up 13% of the population but consume 40% of prescription drugs and 35% of all over the counter drugs.[4] Nearly 92% of older adults have at least one chronic condition, and 77% have at least two.[4] They are the fastest-growing age segment of the population and have the highest average discretionary income of any age group.

For these reasons, health care providers have found the senior market an attractive one to target. However, several problems are associated with segmenting the senior market.[5] One problem is defining the age at which a person is considered a "senior." Marketing researchers have used ages ranging from 50 to 65 years to define the lower end of the senior market. Another problem is that there is not a single senior market segment; seniors make up multiple age segments. Seniors who fall within specific age ranges (e.g., 55 to 64, 65 to 74, 75 to 84, and 85 and over) are more likely to be similar than seniors of all ages. To further complicate matters, people of similar chronological ages may have different physical, psychological, and social ages. Many people do not look or act their age. Seniors with debilitating diseases can appear to be much older than their chronological age, while healthy, active individuals can appear to be much younger. Some seniors may act young, while others may act older than their age.

Literature on the topic indicates that age should not be the sole variable for segmenting the senior market. Bone[5] identified five variables that have been recommended for segmenting the senior market: Discretionary income (the amount of money available for spending after paying for rent, utilities, and other fixed expenses), General level of health, General activity level, Amount of discretionary time not taken up with family, job, and social activities, and degree of social interaction with others.

Geographic Segmentation

Geographic segmentation permits pharmacists to target patients on the basis of location. It can be used to locate lucrative market segments and target those segments with promotional communications. Geographic information is most useful when linked to other segmentation variables such as age, sex, and spending levels.

The U.S. Census Bureau and organizations such as local chambers of commerce provide demographic and other data that can be linked to geographic location. Pharmacists looking for a potential pharmacy location can go online and find data on consumers by location, income, age, and other demographic variables. Competitor locations can be plotted, along with local traffic patterns. Market and economic analyses of the area can also be acquired. Much of this information is available free of charge or for a nominal fee.

Although it might appear that pharmacies are ubiquitous in the US, there are many geographic locations underserved by pharmacists. Availability of pharmacy services in rural settings is still a concern in areas of the United States.[6] Some urban areas of major cities are "pharmacy deserts" (low access communities) where access to prescription medications is difficult.[7] These underserved areas offer opportunities for pharmacists.

PSYCHOGRAPHIC SEGMENTATION

For answering many marketing questions, demographic and geographic data have limited usefulness. These data cannot explain why consumers act the way they do. Age, race, and sex tell little about why a person might select one product over another or be more susceptible to certain promotional messages.

To better understand these issues, marketers conduct psychographic research. Psychographic segmentation is based on the premise that consumer behaviors are influenced by personality, lifestyle, and values. Psychological and sociological research methods, including surveys, focus groups, and personal interviews, are used to identify consumer values, beliefs, and attitudes. Psychographic segmentation is useful for shaping promotional strategies, for product development, and for communication decisions.[8] There are numerous ways to segment markets psychographically.

Personality Segments

Personality segments are based on behavioral traits or personality characteristics such as compulsive, controlling, conservative, socializer, extrovert, and need to achieve. Although heavily studied, personality has not been found to be a consistent predictor of consumer behavior.[8]

Lifestyle Segments

Lifestyle can overlap with personality characteristics but is more useful for segmentation.[8] Lifestyle relates to the activities, interests, and opinions of consumers.[9] Lifestyle segmentation reflects a group's priorities and beliefs about various issues. People's actions (e.g., purchases) tend to be consistent with their interests and opinions.

Lifestyle segmentation has been used to classify senior populations. Moschis[10-12] groups the adults in the United States 55 years of age and over into four segments: health hermits, frail recluses, ailing outgoers, and health indulgers. It was found that these segments could be used to target senior preferences for products, payment methods, and responsiveness to promotional efforts. Shufeldt et al.[13] used lifestyle to identify differences in seniors' nonprescription purchasing behavior. They segmented seniors as follows: family oriented (25.6%), young and secure (19.4%), active retiree (18.1%), self-reliant (20%), and quiet introvert (18.9%). Using these segments, they were able to identify differences in the perceived importance of price, commercial influences, and personal influences on purchases of nonprescription medications.

Segmentation by Values

Values segmentation attempts to identify values upon which people base their lives and day-to-day actions. Values are associated with deeply held beliefs and are key to making important decisions like choosing health care.[8] Knowing which values are important to customer segments can help marketers design and deliver their messages. A pharmacist who wants a patient to adhere to a medication regimen might communicate a different message for a segment that most values security than for a segment that values fun and enjoyment of life.

Psychographic Research and Medications

Psychographic studies have segmented users of pharmaceuticals. In one study of users of cold remedies, four different market segments were identified:[14]

o *Realists* are not overly concerned with protection but are not fatalistic either. They view remedies positively and consider nonprescription therapies to be a convenient health care solution.

o *Authority seekers* are neither fatalists nor stoics about their health. They prefer some stamp of authority on remedies, from either a physician or a pharmacist.

- *Skeptics* have a low concern for health and are the least likely to use medications, including cold remedies.

- *Hypochondriacs* are very concerned with health matters and regard themselves as prone to being affected by all germs and diseases. These people tend to take medications at the onset of the first symptoms of a cold. They seek the expertise and authority of a health care provider for reassurance.

Some researchers combine demographic and psychographic variables to segment markets. Morris et al.[15] segmented users of the AARP (formerly American Association of Retired Persons) pharmacy service into four types of information seekers. "Ambivalent learners" perceived themselves as less than totally healthy and likely to seek out further information about their health and medicines. "Uncertain patients" perceived themselves to be less knowledgeable about their health conditions but in actuality were no less knowledgeable than others. They also believed that adherence to medication regimens would be difficult. "Risk avoiders" used medical information-seeking as a risk-control coping strategy. "Assertively self-reliants" did not feel much need for medical information.

BEHAVIORAL SEGMENTATION

Most individual pharmacists do not have the background in psychometrics, the research skills, or the funding to use psychographic segmentation. Pharmacists may find value in grouping patients into categories based on perceptions and lifestyles. However, a method that is more accessible and easier for the average pharmacist to apply is behavioral segmentation.

Behavioral segmentation uses information about consumer actions and choices to group customers. In a health care environment, it often deals with utilization of health care services and products. Behavioral segmentation criteria might include the type of health insurance or health plan choices available, the frequency of visits to health care providers, self-care habits, prescription drug use, nonprescription and herbal medication use, preventive care behaviors, and level of participation in pharmaceutical care activities.

Many marketers believe segmentation based on actual behavior is particularly valuable because of the strong relationship to future behavior. One argument for using behavioral segmentation in health care is that a relatively small number of people use a disproportionate amount of health care services and products. This phenomenon is described by the *Pareto principle*, which states that approximately 80% of most problems can be attributed to roughly 20% of their potential causes. The Pareto principle would suggest that pharmacists should target the 20% of the market associated with drug misuse, health care spending, and other behaviors, because the potential positive impact will be disproportionately greater than the marketing effort.[16]

The 80–20 rule is shown again and again in health care. A study assessing the applicability of the Pareto principle to address relevant problems of drug therapy found that the ten most frequent symptoms presented at the emergency room were causally involved in 80.0 % of inpatient hospitalizations.[17] in addition, a limited number of drugs and clinical symptoms accounted for a large proportion of ADE at approximately an 80-20 rate.[17]

Segmentation Based on Actual Behavior

Usage

Consumers are often segmented according to the frequency with which they use products and services. Market research firms often provide clients with usage data on a variety of consumer products (e.g., cough and cold medicines) and services (e.g., physician visits) by light, medium, and heavy users. Heavy users are often targeted by marketers, in the belief that persuading one heavy user to use a product or engage in a behavior is better than persuading three or four light users.

This is common in health care where programs seek to reduce emergency department admissions and costs by targeting a small number of "super-user" patients responsible for straining resources by engaging in unnecessary or inappropriate care.[18] In pharmacy, disease management services target populations of patients who have medical conditions that are especially expensive to the health care system. It is believed that attracting patients with diabetes or asthma to a pharmacy will generate greater sales and lead to a greater reduction in overall health care costs than will attracting several people with minor illnesses. *Case management* interventions are also based on usage. Case management attempts to help individual patients with severe health problems navigate efficiently through the health care system. It usually targets individuals who have multiple, chronic, costly conditions.

Heavy users may be a desirable target market, but there are times when targeting moderate or light users or nonusers is better. A large number of patients who are light users or nonusers of health care can indicate latent, unmet demand. Patients who rarely use pharmacist services may actually be those who most need them (e.g., patients who are nonadherent with medications). Their lack of usage may be due to unawareness of their personal pharmaceutical needs, unfamiliarity with the benefits of pharmacist services, or financial or physical barriers to receiving services.

Occasion

Patients can also be grouped according to the occasions or situations in which they make purchasing decisions. Gehrt and Pinto[21] found that consumer selection of pharmacists, physicians, and other health care providers depends on the individual consumer's situation. Consumers were asked to rate the appropriateness of health care choices (e.g., physician, emergency room, pharmacist) in (1) treating major and minor illnesses, (2) at home and on vacation, and (3) for the respondents themselves or for treating family members. The respondents indicated that for major illnesses at home, physicians and emergency rooms were the best alternatives.

For major illnesses away from home on vacation, consumers preferred urgent care centers in addition to physicians and emergency rooms. For minor illnesses at home or on vacation, consumers considered the pharmacist, medicine cabinet, chiropractor, and "do nothing" alternatives to be equally appropriate. There was no difference in responses according to whether treatment was being considered for the respondents themselves or for family members.

User Status and Loyalty

Other behavioral segments address user status and consumer loyalty. User status refers to previous use. It might consider whether consumers are first-time users, former users, repeat users, or potential users. This classification is useful for pharmacists because knowing past use can be helpful in selecting marketing strategies designed to influence future use. Loyalty to a product or service is also a common way of segmenting customers. Marketers often treat customers who have been consistently loyal over time differently from those who have demonstrated partial or no loyalty.

Willingness to Adopt Innovations

Behavioral segmentation can also classify individuals according to their innovativeness and the speed at which they adopt innovations (Figure 12-2).[22]

Innovators are the first to adopt new ideas and products. They usually account for a small percentage of the population (approximately 2.5%). They are characterized as venturesome, eager to try new things, and willing to take risks. They have a broader viewpoint than the typical person, greater education, and the financial capability to absorb failures.

Early adopters are socially connected and influenced by innovators. They typically make up 13.5% of the population and are more likely to influence opinions than any other adopter category. They are sought out for advice, respected by others, and willing to share new ideas through word-of-mouth discussions.

Individuals in the *early majority* are influenced by early adopters, but they are careful, deliberate, and willing to take more time in making decisions. They make up approximately 34% of the population. Although not typically opinion leaders, they are usually well integrated socially.

Late majority individuals make up 34% of the population and are considered cautious and skeptical with regard to innovations. They tend to wait to adopt innovations until social and economic pressures force them to do so.

Laggards make up the last 16% of the population. They are traditional in outlook and look to the past in their decision-making. They are often socially isolated and resist innovations.

This behavioral segmentation scheme shows that adoption of innovations starts with a few individuals. Those innovators share their experiences with others until, over time, the innovation is spread widely throughout the population. The diffusion of innovations model has been used in pharmacy to examine dissemination of patient education It has been used in pharmacy primarily to assess pharmacists' adoption of innovations like patient center services,[23] immunization services,[24] quality improvement strategies,[25] prescribing,[26, 27] and biometric screening services.[28]

Marketers like to identify early adopters within a market.[29, 30] Early adopters are known as *opinion leaders* or *thought leaders* because they are socially connected and likely to influence the diffusion of innovations within a market. Because of their social connections, they are more influential than innovators. Drug companies commonly identify physician thought leaders and work to persuade them to try newly marketed drugs on their patients. The hope is that these thought leaders will adopt the drugs and encourage other physicians to try them.

Figure 12-2 Segmenting customers according to their tendency to adopt innovations.

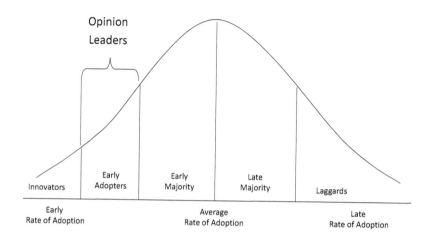

Potential Behavior

A common method of segmentation by potential behavior is to group individuals according to their readiness to buy or act in some desirable manner. Marketers have divided buyer readiness into the following stages: unaware, aware, interest, evaluation, trial, usage, and repeat usage.[31] Knowing the stage of readiness a consumer is in can help improve the effectiveness of marketing interventions. Someone who is unaware or uninterested will likely require a different marketing mix than those in other readiness stages.

Pharmacists often segment patient populations according to readiness to act. One of the most common smoking cessation strategies is based on patients' readiness to change smoking behavior.[32] Five stages of readiness to change (precontemplation, contemplation, preparation, action, and maintenance) require different appeals and strategies.

Mix of Actual and Potential Behavior

In some cases, a combination of actual and potential behaviors is used to segment consumers. Koecheler et al.[33] developed a set of indicators to identify ambulatory pharmacy patients at increased risk for drug-related problems. The following indicators of actual and potential behavior were used to segment their patient population:

1. Patients taking 5 or more medications in their current drug regimen.

2. Patients taking 12 or more medication doses per day.

3. Patients whose medication regimen has changed four or more times in the past 12 months.

4. Patients who have more than three concurrent disease states.

5. Patients who have a history of noncompliance.

6. Patients who are taking drugs that require therapeutic drug monitoring.

Patients with these characteristics were more likely to have drug-related problems. Segmenting patients in this way can help target those patients who might benefit most from pharmacist intervention.

Another segmentation variable being used is patient activation.[19, 20] One tool, called the patient activation measure (PAM) segments consumers into one of four progressively higher activation levels. Each level is associated with distinct self-care behaviors, as well as a wealth of insight into the attitudes, values, motivations, and emotional disposition that drive these behaviors. With these insights, care givers and healthcare organizations can better tailor support and allocate resources more effectively.

BENEFITS SEGMENTATION

Benefits segmentation groups customers according to the specific benefits they seek. It is especially useful for pharmacists because behavior is closely linked to the benefits sought.[34] Some consumers choose their pharmacy on the basis of convenience, because they want to simplify the search or minimize travel time. Others choose pharmacies because of the relationship with their pharmacist or the service received.

In benefits segmentation, it is important to emphasize that customers purchase the core benefits provided by products, not the tangible product. People purchase products and services to meet many different needs and wants—psychological, social, spiritual, and physiological. Pharmacists who can identify and use benefit segments can better serve their patients.

One useful way for pharmacists to group customers is how they trade-off cost and quality. Patrons of pharmacies can be classified into the following four categories:[31]

- *Quality buyers*, who seek the best products and services without regard to cost.
- *Service buyers*, who look for personal and caring services.
- *Value buyers*, who hunt for the best value for the money and expect service to match the price.
- *Economy buyers*, who favor the cheapest alternative.

Consumers of preventive health services have been grouped into the following six benefit segments:[34]

- ○ *Hypochondriac.* People in this segment need and actively seek reassurance that they are healthy. They tend to overuse health services because they believe that doing so will improve their health. They are good customers for vitamins, self-diagnostic kits, and preventive therapies; by using these products, they think they are doing the right thing to maintain health.

- ○ *Health seeker.* Health seekers strive for a long, healthy life and use preventive care as a means to that end. They actively participate in health behaviors such as exercise, healthy eating, and avoidance of smoking, illicit drugs, and alcohol. They actively seek information about healthy practices and preventive services such as health screenings and vaccinations. They also respond to the marketing of health foods.

- ○ *Band-Aider.* Band-Aiders like to brag about how healthy they are. They take great pride in how little they have needed to use health care services. Preventive health care is undesirable to them because it directly contrasts with their self-image of robust health. Band-Aiders seek care only when they are very ill or injured.

- ○ *Do not bug me.* People in this segment use negative health behavior such as overeating, smoking, and drug and alcohol use to cope with the daily stresses of life. They avoid preventive health care, although they may be the segment most likely to benefit from it.

- ○ *Follower.* Followers seek the guidance of others for preventive practices. They might seek advice from friends, family members, or health care professionals. They tend to do what others recommend but can be skeptical that preventive health care will bring about the promised improvements in health. They are more likely to put off health care until they get sick. They are unlikely to use vitamins and preventive remedies or to attend health screenings unless it is recommended by others.

- ○ *Self-sufficient.* These independent, self-reliant individuals tend to be skeptical of traditional health care and prefer to treat themselves with home remedies and nonprescription medications. Their skepticism often comes from previous negative experiences with health care.

MARKETING IN ACTION

Looking for Jobs to Be Done

Ted Levitt, a famous marketer, once commented that consumers buy ¼ inch holes, not electric drills with ¼ inch drill bits. Recently, Clay Christensen has argued that consumers "hire" products and services to fulfill specific jobs. Both Levitt and Christensen are speaking about the importance of identifying and serving the benefits sought by customers.

Benefits segmentation examines the problems faced by customers instead of the tangible product or intangible program being offered to them. Christensen's job-to-be-done examines benefits from the customer's viewpoint.[35] It looks at:

The functional job - describes how the consumer gets a specific task done or achieves a goal

The emotional job - describes how the customer feels or wants to feel.

The social job - describes how the customer wants to be perceived by others.

The job associated with a mother's visit to the pharmacy to fill a prescription antibiotic for a child might consist of the following jobs:

The functional job - "I want to cure my child's infection."

The emotional job - "I want to protect my child from danger and feel like I am a good mother."

The social job - "I want others to see that I am a good mother who does the right thing for her child."

Pharmacists can help patient with fundamental jobs in their lives which consist primarily of (1) helping diagnose what is wrong, (2) giving a solution, and (3) helping them maintain their health.[36] Pharmacists do not have to do what they have always done to fulfill these fundamental jobs. If fact, changes in health care and technology almost ensure that the old way will not work much longer.

New business models need to be developed to help serve patient jobs-to-be-done. Peter Drucker was famously quoted as saying, "The customer rarely buys what the business thinks it sells him." The goal for pharmacists in benefits segmentation is to spend time and effort finding out what customers really want, not what we think they want.

Source: References [35,36]

SEGMENTATION FOR THE PRACTICING PHARMACIST

It is important for pharmacists to remember that the goal of segmentation is to help identify and predict consumer tendencies to act in specific ways. This information can then be used to influence consumer behavior in some manner. The value of segmentation variables is their ability to act as surrogates for behavior. The information has little value to a marketer if it cannot be put to use to predict and influence behavior.

Researching the Market

In order to segment a market, pharmacists need to conduct research into their patients' needs and wants. There are several marketing research methods that any pharmacist can use, many of them at little or no cost.

Talk with patients. One-to-one conversations provide insight into customer needs. Good pharmacists talk with patients about their lives and problems to help identify better ways to serve them. Motivational interviewing can help uncover opportunities to help.

Invite a group of patients to chat about pharmacy services. This can be done in a formal focus group or less formally with a group of people sitting around a table. In focus groups, people are encouraged to share information they might not share in one-to-one conversations. Pharmacists can pay marketing research companies to conduct focus groups, or they can conduct them on their own.

Conduct surveys. Surveys are useful for gathering information and statistics about a large group of customers. One problem with surveys is getting people to respond to them. The key to increasing the response rate is to make it easy to respond. Surveys should be as short as possible, easy to read, and accessible. Many businesses place customer surveys on 5 by 10 inch cards and locate them near the point of service. Short internet surveys can also be used.

Read the pharmacy and health care literature. There are many articles describing important trends, new developments in the profession, and ideas for segmenting patient populations.

Use the Internet. Internet search engines permit pharmacists to search the world for information without leaving their chairs. The key is to differentiate information that is useful from the useless.

Mine patient data files. Pharmacists can analyze patient purchasing and usage patterns through scanner data or patient medication profiles. The data can be used to identify behavioral patterns that might be of use in marketing.

Observe how customers shop. Answer the following questions, "What do they do while waiting for services? What do they purchase? How do they purchase? How much time do they take? On what components of the package or promotional material do they focus?"

Test-market ideas. Before offering a service on a full time basis, hold a one-day event to test whether customers like the service and what they like or dislike about it. Consider expanding it to one day each week or full-time at one store in a chain.

USING SEGMENTATION IN PRACTICE

Individual pharmacists can use segmentation to target specific customer groups for their services. Here are the steps:

1. Identify key market segments within your practice. Start with easy-to-define segments such as customers with different disease states, large numbers of prescriptions, or specific needs. As experience is gained, new segments may be identified.

2. Learn as much as you can about the segments in which you are interested. Try to identify how information in the published literature relates to your patients.

3. Describe a typical person (i.e., persona) in a market segment. Commonly used in marketing, personas are fictional characters created to represent different customers of interest based upon demographic, benefit, behavioral, attitudinal, or other demographic variables. Personas are often used to generate better questions and discussions about customer segment needs and wants by personalizing the segments.

4. Determine the desirability of each segment. This can be done by calculating the average lifetime value of customers in the segment, the number of customers in the segment, or some other measure.

5. Select those segments on which you wish to focus and create a written plan for each segment. Describe what specific actions will be taken to meet the needs of customers in each segment.

6. Establish a budget for each segment. The budget should include allocations of both money and time. Explicit understanding of the costs involved will help improve the chances of success.

7. Develop measures for the success of targeting efforts (e.g., sales volume, number of repeat visits).

8. Choose a future date when you will reassess your marketing efforts.

SUMMARY

It is important to choose segmentation variables carefully. Select only one or two segmentation criteria to begin with; more than a few can be hard to keep track of. Make certain that the segments are based on clear marketing objectives and a solid knowledge of your customer base.

MARKETING IN ACTION

How Target Got into Hot Water Using Segmentation

Target, like all major retailers, collects intimate data about customers and their consumption behaviors. They use that information to figure out customers like, what they need, and which coupons to use to encourage future business. Target got into trouble by using poor judgment in their data-mining of customers. [37] Specifically, they started sending coupons for baby items to customers who may not have shared details about a pregnancy with family members.

Reportedly, an angry father visited a Target saying, " My daughter got this in the mail!", showing a manager a mailer addressed to the man's daughter and containing advertisements for maternity clothing, nursery furniture and pictures of smiling infants. The father said, "She's still in high school, and you're sending her coupons for baby clothes and cribs? Are you trying to encourage her to get pregnant?"

What happened is that Target was able to accurately diagnose the daughter's pregnancy through purchasing history of things like unscented lotion; supplements like calcium, magnesium and zinc; scent-free soap and extra-big bags of cotton balls; hand sanitizers; and washcloths. Using approximately 25 products, Target was able to assign shoppers a "pregnancy prediction" score that might trigger flyers and coupons to be sent to a person's address.

A few days later, the father had to call up the manager with an apology. The abashed father said, "I had a talk with my daughter. It turns out there's been some activities in my house I haven't been completely aware of. She's due in August."

This story was widely reported in the news and caused Target to suspend their targeting program, at least temporarily. It gave them a public relations black eye that they did not need.

Source: Reference[37]

Reference List

(1) LaFleur EK, Taylor SE. Women's health centers and specialized services: segmentation strategies can be effective in targeting some female health care consumers. Journal of Health Care Marketing, 1996;16(3):16-24.

(2) Anon. Aging boomers, new medicines draw men into health spotlight. Drug Store News 2000.

(3) Silverstein MJ, Sayre K. The female economy. Harvard Business Review 2009;87(9):46-53.

(4) American Society of Consultant Pharmacists. ASCP Fact Sheet. 1-31-2015. 1-31-2015.

(5) Fitzgerald Bone P. Identifying mature segments. Journal of consumer Marketing 1991;8(4):19-32.

(6) Casey MM, Klingner J, Moscovice I. Pharmacy services in rural areas: Is the problem geographic access or financial access? The Journal of Rural Health 2002;18(3):467-477.

(7) Qato DM, Daviglus ML, Wilder J, Lee T, Qato D, Lambert B. 'Pharmacy deserts' are prevalent in Chicago's predominantly minority communities, raising medication access concerns. Health Aff (Millwood) 2014;33(11):1958-1965.

(8) Yankelovich D, Meer D. Rediscovering market segmentation. Harvard Business Review 2006;84(2):122.

(9) Plummer JT. The concept and application of life style segmentation. the journal of marketing 1974;33-37.

(10) George PM, Leah B. Marketing pharmaceutical and cosmetic products to the mature market. Intl J of Pharm & Health Mrkt 2013;7(4):357-373.

(11) Moschis GP, Friend SB. Segmenting the preferences and usage patterns of the mature consumer health-care market. Intl J of Pharm & Health Mrkt 2008;2(1):7-21.

(12) Moschis GP, Bellenger DN, Curasi CF. What influences the mature consumer? Mark Health Serv 2003;23(4):16-21.

(13) Shufeldt L, Oates B, Vaught B. Is lifestyle an important factor in the purchase of OTC drugs by the elderly? Journal of consumer Marketing 1998;15(2):111-124.

(14) Ziff R. Psychographics for market segmentation. Journal of Advertising Research 1971;11(2):3-9.

(15) Morris LA, Tabak ER, Olins NJ. A segmentation analysis of prescription drug information-seeking motives among the elderly. Journal of Public Policy & Marketing 1992;115-125.

(16) Wansink B, Park SB. Methods and measures that profile heavy users. Journal of Advertising Research 2000;40(2000):61-72.

(17) Muller F, Dormann H, Pfistermeister B et al. Application of the Pareto principle to identify and address drug-therapy safety issues. Eur J Clin Pharmacol 2014;70(6):727-736.

(18) Ku BS, Fields JM, Santana A, Wasserman D, Borman L, Scott KC. The Urban Homeless: Super-users of the Emergency Department. Popul Health Manag 2014;17(6):366-371.

(19) Hendriks M, Rademakers J. Relationships between patient activation, disease-specific knowledge and health outcomes among people with diabetes; a survey study. BMC Health Services Research 2014;14:-393.

(20) Heller A, Elliott MN, Haviland AM, Klein DJ, Kanouse DE. Patient activation status as a predictor of patient experience among Medicare beneficiaries. Medical care 2009;47(8):850-857.

(21) Gehrt KC, Pinto MB. Assessing the viability of situationally driven segmentation opportunities in the health care market. Hospital & health services administration 1992;38(2):243-265.

(22) Rogers EM. Diffusion of innovations. Simon and Schuster; 2010.

(23) Pronk MC, Blom LT, Jonkers R, Rogers EM, Bakker A, de Blaey KJ. Patient oriented activities in Dutch community pharmacy: diffusion of innovations. Pharm World Sci 2002;24(4):154-161.

(24) Westrick SC. Forward and backward transitions in pharmacy-based immunization services. Res Social Adm Pharm 2010;6(1):18-31.

(25)Sorensen AV, Bernard SL. Accelerating what works: using qualitative research methods in developing a change package for a learning collaborative. Jt Comm J Qual Patient Saf 2012;38(2):89-95.

(26) Paudyal V, Hansford D, Cunningham S, Stewart D. Over-the-counter prescribing and pharmacists' adoption of new medicines: diffusion of innovations. Res Social Adm Pharm 2013;9(3):251-262.

(27) Makowsky MJ, Guirguis LM, Hughes CA, Sadowski CA, Yuksel N. Factors influencing pharmacists' adoption of prescribing: qualitative application of the diffusion of innovations theory. Implement Sci 2013;8:109.

(28) Teeter BS, Braxton-Lloyd K, Armenakis AA, Fox BI, Westrick SC. Adoption of a biometric screening service in community pharmacies: a qualitative study. J Am Pharm Assoc (2003) 2014;54(3):258-266.

(29) Fugh-Berman A, Ahari S. Following the script: how drug reps make friends and influence doctors. PLoS Medicine 2007;4(4):e150.

(30) Berwick DM. Disseminating innovations in health care. JAMA 2003;289(15):1969-1975.

(31) Kotler P. Marketing Management: Analysis, Planning, and Control. 4th ed. Engelwood Cliffs, NJ: Prentice Hall; 1980.

(32) Kennedy DT, Small RE. Development and implementation of a smoking cessation clinic in community pharmacy practice. J Am Pharm Assoc (Wash) 2002;42(1):83-92.

(33) Koecheler JA, Abramowitz PW, Swim SE, Daniels CE. Indicators for the selection of ambulatory patients who warrant pharmacist monitoring. American Journal of Health-System Pharmacy 1989;46(4):729-732.

(34) John J, Miaoulis G. A model for understanding benefit segmentation in preventive health care. Health care management review 1992;17(2):21-32.

(35) Developing Consumer Solutions Using Jobs to Be Done. 2015. Innosight. 2-1-2015.

(36) Wanamaker B. Satisfying the patient's jobs-to-be-done. 10-3-2013. Clayton Christensen Institute for Disruptive Innovation. 2-1-2015.

(37) Hill K. How Target figured out a teen girl was pregnant before her father did. Forbes, Inc 2012.

Chapter Questions

1. What is the purpose of segmenting pharmacy markets? Compare and contrast segmentation, targeting, and positioning.

2. List the characteristics of a desirable market segment.

3. Comment on why pharmacists may not want to target the largest segment in markets.

4. What demographic variables in Table 12-1 are most associated with prescription drug use in general? Oral antibiotics? Birth control products?

5. What problems are associated with targeting the senior market? What other variables within the senior market are useful in segmentation? How might these variables affect drug consumption and use?

6. How might an understanding of psychographics help pharmacists design promotional messages to different patient market segments?

7. What is the Pareto principle? How does it relate to behavioral segmentation?

8. Should pharmacists target "light" or "heavy" users of prescription medicines? Why?

9. Should pharmacists segment patients for medication therapy management services care according to disease state or general health care needs (i.e., case management)?

PART V

Pricing and Marketing Communication

CHAPTER 13

PRICING PHARMACIST SERVICES
Co-authored by Norman Carroll

Objectives

After studying this chapter, the reader should be able to

- Explain why pricing is an important part of marketing pharmacy products and services.
- Discuss how pricing relates to other elements of the marketing mix
- List and discuss the effects of consumer-related factors, competition, pharmacy objectives, and costs on pricing decisions
- Calculate the cost of providing a pharmacist service
- Explain the relationships among price, cost, and demand for a pharmacist service
- List and explain the steps involved in one strategy for pricing pharmacist services

Price is what you pay. Value is what you get.

-Warren Buffett

THE SCIENCE AND ART OF PRICING

Of the 4P's, price is the only element of the marketing mix that generates revenue for pharmacies. It helps determine the revenue associated with the provision of product, place, and promotion. Effective pricing determines the success of a service, product, or business.

There is a science and art to pricing pharmacy products and services. Social sciences like economics and consumer psychology provide clues to the science. The art of pricing occurs for situations that are not easily explained by science. For instance, theories are often weak predictors of actual behavior, so marketers need to rely on experience and hunches in setting prices. Marketers must walk a tightrope of charging enough to make a profit but not charging too much to be seen as unfairly gouging customers. The key is to persuade customers that what is being offered is worth what is being charged.

There is no magic process that says, "If I do this, customers will do that". Therefore, most pharmacists rely on cost accounting principles to set prices for pharmacist services.[1-8] This chapter will go beyond cost based pricing and explore other variables in generating revenue to support pharmacist services.

Several important definitions need to be understood when talking about pricing:

- *Price* is the amount paid by a party in a transaction in return for goods or services. A price may be paid in money, goods (i.e., barter), physical or mental effort, or any other form of compensation for what is received.

- *Compensation* is payment for doing a job like MTM services.

- *Reimbursement* is paying someone back an amount equal to what that person has invested in terms of money and effort. It is different from compensation which is not directly linked to what has been invested. When speaking about professional pharmacist services like MTM, the preferred terminology is compensation, not reimbursement.

- A *charge* is what a seller asks to be paid or compensated for doing a job. It differs from compensation which is the amount actually paid. This is an important distinction because the amount charged by health care providers is often much more than what is actually compensated for by customers like health insurance companies.

- A *cost* is the amount of resources needed to produce goods or services. It consists of inputs like employee salaries, facilities, overhead, materials, and other production costs.

- *Revenue* is the total amount of income (i.e., money) received by an entity (e.g., pharmacy) from all sources. Revenue might come from compensation from services, sales of merchandise, grants and donations from organizations, or any other source of income.

Understanding how these terms differ is important for pharmacists who want to generate sufficient revenue to survive in business. Customers care little what a pharmacist service costs - only what they have to pay for it. And pharmacists can charge high prices for services, but compensation only occurs when customers pay.

It is equally important to emphasize that costs can be nonmonetary. Many "free services" offered by pharmacists are not perceived as free in the minds of patients. A free medication adherence program, for example, requires patients to actively participate in their care. They may need to change habits, receive reminder phone calls, track their own medication use, and do other things that take physical and mental effort. If that effort is perceived as too expensive in the minds of the patients, they may choose to quit taking medications as directed. Clear understanding of all of the costs paid by the customer is crucial in pricing pharmacist services.

MARKETING IN ACTION

All Bargain Shoppers are Not Alike

Everyone loves a bargain. However, all bargain shoppers are not the same.

Many bargain shoppers consider more than just price in their decisions. Some are willing to pay higher prices under the right conditions. They might pay for more and still feel they are getting a bargain if the overall service experience meets their expectations. Understanding the tradeoffs made for price in shopping is important in helping pharmacists tailor deals and discounts for the right audience and in the right channels.

A survey of 25,000 U.S. adults identified six types of bargain shoppers.[9] Experian, the agency that conducted the study, categorized the wide range of attitudes, behaviors and motivations of deal-seekers into the following categories:

1. *Offline deal-seekers.* These shoppers are typically over age 55 and love to find deals in stores. They head straight to the clearance rack when they enter a store but are unwilling to travel far to shop. They are highly social with many different groups of friends, but their influence in the digital domain is limited as they are less likely than average to engage in social media. This segment is also less likely to use the Internet to plan shopping trips or compare prices.

2. *Deal thrillers.* Deal thrillers love getting a deal but are also loyal to specific brands. Their thrill for the deal does not equal a thrill for

coupons. They are less likely, in general, to use coupons to get deals.

3. *Deal takers*. Deal takers are highly educated and affluent consumers who do not seek deals but will accept one if offered. Promotions targeted at deal takers must be easily accessible online and offline. They will change behaviors given the right sale or coupon.

4. *Deal indifferents*. Deal indifferents are the largest deal seeking segment of the population, and they do not respond to deals. Most only shop when they have a specific need, and coupons are wasted on them.

5. *Deal-seeker influentials*. Influentials constantly look for the best online, offline and mobile deals. They tend to be young, highly educated, socially active consumers who love shopping but think paying full price is for suckers. They trust the information they see about products on social media and often respond to online advertising on social platforms. Active on the Internet and social media, their recommendations are influential with individuals within their social circles.

6. *Deal rejectors*. Deal rejectors hate shopping, preferring convenience over everything. They tend to be male, older, and willing to pay more for convenience.

CONSIDERATIONS IN PRICING

The *perspective* of customers or other decision makers is important in pricing pharmacist services and goods. From the patient's perspective, the perceived price of a drug might consist of an out-pocket co-payment and transportation to a pharmacy. From the perspective of an employer who pays for employee insurance coverage, the perceived price might be the compensation paid for the drug itself and any pharmacy services provided with the drug. Pharmacists need to understand the perspective of who pays, how much is paid, and what exactly is being paid for when pricing their goods and services.

The *market* being served is also crucial in pricing. Pharmacists typically serve up to three different markets: consumer, institutional, and governmental. Pricing in consumer markets requires an understanding of consumer psychology. Pharmacists who price consumer goods and services must take into account the idiosyncratic thought processes and behaviors of consumers which are more subjective and often have a peculiar logic to objective observers. On the other hand, pricing for institutional and governmental markets requires insight into organizational decision making. Often acceptance of a price depends on a pharmacist making an objective business case to purchasers. This means identifying key decision makers and communicating how a pharmacist service or product can provide a positive return on investment (ROI).

The *product or service* offered for sale can determine pricing strategies. Pricing is influenced by whether pharmacists are offering non-durable goods, durable goods, or services.

- *Non-durable goods.* Most pharmacies generate the majority of their revenue from non-durable goods like drugs, bandages, and other things that are purchased and consumer frequently. Most non-durable goods are priced slightly above their cost to produce in order to generate sales volume. The pricing strategy is to produce many small profits on a high volume of sales. Specialty medicines are an exception to the typical non-durable good because they can be quite expensive -- often over $100,000 per year of therapy.

- *Durable goods.* Durable goods are tangible products that last through repeated use. In pharmacies, durable goods include medical devices like glucometers and durable medical equipment like wheelchairs and orthotics. These goods typically require pharmacists to train patients and provide support in their use.

- *Services.* Services are intangible and not durable. They are more difficult to price than merchandise because customers have difficulty recognizing and appreciating the value they provide. Pricing services requires different strategies than that of durable and non-durable goods.

The *buyer's power* to influence prices is a big issue in pricing pharmacy services. Buyers who have power can force sellers to offer a price which the buyer feels is acceptable. Porter[10] states that a buyer's power depends on the following characteristics of markets:

1. *The level of rivalry between competitors.* The more competitors who are fighting for buyers, the less flexibility sellers have to raise prices. Intense competition in retail pharmacy markets have driven down the service component of the drug prices.

2. *The ease with which new sellers can enter a market.* The harder it is for sellers to enter a market, the easier it is for those who remain to charge high prices. High barriers-to-entry make it difficult for low price sellers to enter and take market share from high price sellers. Prior to the 1960's, many states only allowed pharmacists to own pharmacies, giving pharmacists the ability to charge higher prices and make greater profit margins on prescriptions sold. Changes in state laws permitting pharmacy ownership by nonpharmacists and corporations have lowered market barriers and lead to steep declines in pharmacist pricing flexibility.

3. *The availability of substitutes.* The more substitutes for a seller's products and services, the more difficult it is for sellers to charge higher prices. For example, unique new drugs are often able to command high prices from purchasers until substitutes can be found. When possible, health systems attempt to generate price competition for more expensive brand name

pharmaceuticals with therapeutic substitution policies that allow pharmacists to automatically substitute therapeutically similar but not generically equivalent competitors.

PRICING AND STRATEGY

A business's general strategy influences the pricing it uses. Businesses that use low cost strategies, like WalMart which is consistently recognized as being the leader in low costs, compete by undercutting the prices of competitors. Winning large numbers of customers away from competitors makes up for lower profit margins and enables WalMart to remain profitable. Profits are then invested into finding ways to lower prices even more, like buying new systems of automation and inventory control.

Some cost based strategies focus on lowering the price of drugs (e.g., "We offer 4-dollar prescriptions."). Pharmacies that focus on lowering the cost of drugs are at a continual competitive disadvantage to low cost leaders. The cost advantages of low cost leaders allow them to profit at price levels that are unprofitable to low cost followers. Consequently, low cost followers either find some other way to make up lost profits, differentiate themselves on something other than cost, or go out of business.

Some pharmacies reframe the low cost argument more broadly by focusing on lowering costs to the entire health care supply chain (e.g., "Our MTM services are more cost effective for treating most chronic conditions"). They try to make a case to payers that pharmacists add value by improving medication adherence, coordinating care, promoting health, and reducing avoidable emergency department visits, doctors visits, hospitalizations, and nursing home admissions. As described in Chapter 5, total health care costs are determined by the following equation:

$$Total\ Health\ Care\ Costs = f(P,V,I)$$

P = Price (or cost) of services/products for all individuals served
V = Volume or amount of services/products for all individuals served
I = Intensity of health care provided

Pharmacists can make a cost based argument that increasing the intensity of medication therapy services provided by pharmacists can lower total health care costs by (1) helping patients substitute lower priced drugs through generic or therapeutic substitution, (2) helping patients substitute lower priced services like immunizations and diagnostic testing, (3) reducing the volume of unnecessary or inappropriate medication use, and (4) reducing the volume of unavoidable negative health events by helping patients take their drugs correctly.

MARKETING IN ACTION

Charging for What You Are Worth

A new graduate revealed to her mentor that she did not feel comfortable asking patients to pay for her professional services. The mentor shared the following story based upon a famous legend about the time that Pablo Picasso, the famous artist, was sketching in the park and approached by a bold woman.

The woman exclaimed, "It's you — Picasso, the great artist! Oh, you must sketch my portrait! I insist."

So Picasso agreed to sketch her. After studying her for a moment, he used a single pencil stroke to create her portrait. He handed the women his work of art.

"It's perfect!" she gushed. "You managed to capture my essence with one stroke, in one moment. Thank you! How much do I owe you?"

"Five thousand dollars," Picasso replied.

"But, what?" the woman sputtered. "How could you want so much money for this picture? It only took you a second to draw it!"

To which Picasso responded, "Madame, it took me my entire life."

With a wry smile, the new graduate said, "What you are saying is that compensation is determined by the quality of the work provided to produce that effort plus all of the education and training that went into developing the ability to provide that quality. Correct?"

The mentor replied, "I couldn't have said it better."

Pharmacies use cost based arguments to promote specialty pharmacy services that control the overall costs of patients who use expensive, complex medications that may cost tens of thousands of dollars per course of therapy. Pharmacies also use cost based appeals to be compensated for medication therapy management, disease management programs, vaccination services, and most other forms of clinical services offered by pharmacists.

Instead of focusing on providing low cost medications, they make a business case with payers that spending more on pharmacist services will save costs in other areas of the health care supply chain. This is much different from pricing a bottle of aspirin or a tube of hydrocortisone ointment.

PRICE AND BRANDING

Pricing is closely linking with branding. A strong brand can yield a higher price. The brand is a promise that tells buyers that "if you buy this brand, it will be worth the extra you pay for it." A weak pharmacy brand is at a pricing disadvantage to strong brands.

How can pharmacists improve their brand and garner higher prices? This is achieved by having a strong story surrounding the brand and clearly communicating to buyers the time and effort that pharmacists spend in bringing extra value to the customer and the fairness of the price given the amount of time, energy, and care that went into delivering it.

Purchase decisions are influenced by the actual prices charged and consumers' perceptions of the seller's price image.[20] A consumer's perception of how a pharmacy's offerings compares with other pharmacies can influence (1) how consumers evaluate prices of individual items, (2) the perceived fairness of those prices, (3) the decision to purchase, and (4) the quantity of items purchased.[20]

Therefore, prices of individual products and services affect and are affected by the overall price image of a pharmacy. This means that price setting should consider the reciprocal impact of prices on services and services on prices. Table 13-1 illustrates the link between price and brand image is its suggestions for getting compensated for professional services.

Table 13-1 Suggestions for Getting Compensated for Professional Services

1. Let customers know that you do more than fill prescriptions. Pharmacists need to build on their earned public trust and demonstrate their expertise in providing patient care services.

2. Educate physicians about your services. Physicians' recommendations to use your service can positively influence a patient's decision to do so.

3. Believe in the value of your services and have the confidence to request payment. Giving away services for free sends a signal to the patient that your services are not valuable. Avoid the habit of giving free services.

4. It is easier to lower fees than raise them, so be cautious about waiving fees to promote sales during the initial launch of a medication therapy service. Doing so may train patients to resist paying fees in the future.

5. If a program is introduced at a discounted fee, make sure that your promotional messaging makes it clear to patients that the special lower rate is for a limited time only and communicate what the cost will be after the limited time

promotion ends.

6.   Brush up on basic sales techniques. Pharmacists need to sell themselves and their services to succeed.

7.   Don't apologize for charging for your medication therapy services. Pharmacists who lack confidence in communicating the value of their services send the wrong message to potential patients. Speak with confidence about your services and fees to convey their value and importance to potential purchasers.

Source: Reference[21]

HOW TO PRICE PHARMACIST SERVICES

One of the most important questions to answer in every business is, "What price should I charge for my services?" The correct answer should be "as much as you need to generate revenue objectives." Depending on the marketing strategy of the business, the price for a service might be set high to generate maximum revenue, set competitively to equal what competitors are offering, or set low to attract new customers. Price setting in pharmacy should be a function of what customers will pay, the amount of revenue desired and needed, what competitors are charging, the portfolio of services and products being offered, and the other variables of the marketing mix.

Step 1. Set price objectives

A pharmacy's pricing should be consistent with its overall revenue objectives. The objective of most pharmacies is to maximize overall revenues of the pharmacy's portfolio of products and services. To do this, the pharmacist must set prices low enough to attract and retain customers but high enough to generate sufficient revenues to cover the costs of doing business plus an additional profit.

Prices for individual products and services, in retail businesses, are typically set using a portfolio strategy (see Chapter Five Marketing Strategies). A portfolio is all the products and services offered by a business (e.g., a community pharmacy), and portfolio pricing considers the overall contribution of each product and service to the business's revenue. The purpose of portfolio pricing in competitive markets is to choose the right mix of prices for products and services to maximize revenue. In community pharmacy, the conventional strategy is to make money on non-prescription merchandise and price pharmacy services low to get people into the store.

Portfolio pricing requires pharmacists to do several things. The first is to identify the primary target markets served by the pharmacy. Knowing things like their medical conditions, service preferences, income levels, insurance coverage, and ability to pay will influence pricing decisions. Then pharmacists should inventory current sources of revenue. Pharmacies with minimal front-end merchandise will need to price pharmacy services high enough to cover the costs of doing business. In contrast, a pharmacy with a profitable front-end may be able to offer services at prices that only cover some business costs.

Finally, pharmacists need to set prices based upon sales and revenue targets for the overall portfolio (not just the individual product or service). For example, a new pharmacy might have the objective of rapidly building sales volume and revenue. To meet this objective, the pharmacy would offer low prices to attract business. This sacrifices short-term profits in order to build sales and revenue quickly: a strategy called *penetration pricing*. Penetration pricing is preferred in situations where demand is highly elastic (i.e., consumers are price sensitive), where there is strong competition, and where increased volume leads to economies of scale.

Some pharmacies use loss leaders to increase sales and profits. Loss leaders are typically high-demand products or services for which prices are well known. A *loss leader strategy* involves selling these products at or below cost in order to attract consumers into the pharmacy. The pharmacy expects these consumers to also buy other, more profitable, goods and services. Loss leader pricing differs from penetration pricing in that the former offers low prices only on a few selected products in a product portfolio whereas the latter typically offers a low price on a single product or service with the goal of adjusting prices in the future after it is more widely adopted.

A variation on the loss leader approach is a *freemium strategy*.[11] Freemium is a newly coined term that links the words free and premium. Freemium describes a business model that offers a product or service for free, while promoting a complementary product at a positive price. Pharmaceutical companies use a freemium strategy when offering "free" samples of brand medications to physicians. The strategy is to encourage future purchases of the drugs once the free samples run out.

Other pharmacies have the objective of serving only those consumers who are willing to pay higher prices. This is a *price-skimming strategy*. It usually requires offering a service that is not widely available or offering a level of overall service that other pharmacies cannot or choose not to provide. Many specialist physicians and lawyers use a price-skimming strategy; they serve only those consumers who are willing to pay for their higher levels of training and expertise.

Price skimming often occurs when pricing new products or services. This is done to maximize profits on a highly desirable offering as quickly as possible. It is common when there are a substantial number of price-insensitive consumers and few substitutes for the product or service. Pharmaceutical companies usually use price skimming when introducing unique patent-protected medications, especially first products in a new therapeutic class. Examples include each new innovation for treating Hepatitis C which is more expensive than the last and can reach upwards of $100,000.

Businesses that introduce products and services at a skimming price typically lower the price over time. They do this to attract additional business by serving more price-sensitive markets and respond to low price competitors. This only occurs if another innovation does not make it obsolete in the market.

Many pharmacies use *competitive pricing* as their primary strategy. In this situation, a pharmacy prices products and services at the same level as the competition. This is common for a pharmacy that faces strong competitors and has no distinct competitive advantage. In this circumstance, setting higher prices would drive customers to competitors (i.e., higher prices lead to lower demand in competitive markets), and setting lower prices could start a price war with competitors. In competitive and undifferentiated markets, a pharmacy might be quite happy to share part of the market with competitors with competitive pricing.

Cost-plus pricing is typical for pharmacist services.[1, 2, 6] Cost-plus pricing occurs when a pharmacy sets price to break-even with the cost of providing the service (plus a small profit). All costs in the production of the service are calculated. Then a projection is made on how many services can and will be provided in a time period. Next a price is set for each unit of service which will cover the costs plus a profit. For instance, if a MTM program costs $30,000 to set up and maintain over a year and 300 MTM sessions can be provided during that year, the break even cost to provide each MTM session would be $100 (excluding profit). With cost-plus pricing, there is an incentive to reduce costs as much as possible in order to allow services to be offered at lower, more competitive prices.

Variable cost pricing (also called marginal cost pricing) sets a price that covers the variable cost of production while ignoring fixed and overhead costs. The goal is to contribute toward the costs of running the pharmacy but not cover the total cost. This strategy needs to be part of an overall portfolio strategy where revenue from a "cash cow" (see chapter 5) covers the fixed and overhead costs of a "star" or a "question mark". Variable cost pricing might occur for professional services that are offered in a market that will not accept a price that covers total costs of production. As long as the service covers its variable costs, it can contribute to the business's mission.

Value-based pricing centers upon the value of a product or service to a buyer exclusive of production cost. Value-based pricing considers perceived value to the buyer, available alternatives, and willingness-to-pay. The buyer will purchase a product or service only if it is believed that its value exceeds its price. Whether the buyer believes this depends on a number of factors:

- a buyer's perceived need,
- a buyer's willingness-to-pay
- the quality of the product or service relative to alternatives,
- the accessibility and convenience of the product or service,
- the persuasiveness of communications about value, and
- availability of other providers (i.e., competitors).

Value-based pricing relies not only on price, but on all elements of the marketing mix. This has several important implications for setting prices. First, pharmacists should understand the perceived value of any offering to the buyer. In value-based pricing, pharmacists' beliefs are irrelevant; only the buyer's opinion is important. Second, the price selected must be consistent with other elements of the marketing mix. The service itself and the manner in which it is provided, promoted, and delivered must convey the same message as the price about the service's value. Third, cost is not the only, or even the primary, factor in determining the appropriate price. Consumers' perceptions of the service and of the competition are the primary driver of price. The optimal price for a service will be what the customer is willing to pay for it.

Value-base pricing is becoming more common strategy for pharmaceutical companies[12-14] and health insurance.[15-17] It is also argued as necessary for reforming health care in the US.[18, 19] Value-based pricing in pharmacy uses pharmacoeconomic analysis of health care alternatives to establish prices commensurate with the overall value provided. For example, a pharmacist-managed anticoagulation clinic that saves significantly more hospitalization costs than alternative health care options can potentially price services independent of the costs of providing them.

Step 2. Estimate costs

The price of a pharmacist service must be sufficient to cover all or a portion of service costs, product costs, and net profit. Service costs include salaries, rent and utilities, depreciation, and insurance required to provide the service. Product costs are the tangible products that accompany the service which include medications and drug packaging. Finally, there is profit (also called net income).

Product cost is often the largest component in the dispensing of medications because drugs are expensive, especially for specialty medicines. Average product costs per prescription dispensed hovers around $100. Service cost associated with each prescription dispensed averages only approximately $15.

However, service costs can also be substantial depending on the intensity of services provided and the type of service. For example, medication therapy management services are often provided independently of any product. Actually, some MTM providers have no product costs because they are consulting companies (i.e., pure services).

Profit is a smaller but important part of the costs of doing business. If a pharmacy business is to earn a satisfactory profit, its prices must cover its costs plus some surplus for net income. This is more complicated than it may seem, because costs, sales volume, and price are interrelated. Changes in one usually result in changes in the others. In fact, low prices set for one component (e.g., dispensing fee) might be made up by increasing the price charged for another (e.g., dispensed medicine).

For example, a pharmacist who offers a smoking cessation clinic in a pharmacy might estimate the costs of providing patients with nicotine gum and behavioral counseling to help them stop smoking. The product cost for each course of treatment might be whatever the pharmacy charges for an 8-week supply of nicotine gum and the service cost may consist of the pharmacist's salary for an estimated 5 hours of counseling over the course of 12 weeks. Additional costs might come from software programs to support the clinic, time spent training personnel, and advertising. To accurately calculate service costs, a manager must understand several different kinds of costs and how they are related.

Startup and Operating Costs

Costs of new programs are usually separated into startup and operating costs. Startup costs are one-time costs associated with beginning the service. Startup costs for a smoking cessation clinic might include costs of remodeling, training, and purchases of technology. These costs might be covered by a one-time payment of cash from a grant or other investment, or they might be built into costs of the service as a capital investment. Operating costs are the daily program expenses which fall into fixed and variable costs.

Fixed and Variable Costs

The total costs of starting up and operating a service can be broken into fixed and variable costs. *Fixed costs* are those that remain the same regardless of the volume of services and products provided. Building rent is a fixed cost. No matter how high the pharmacy's sales go during a given year, the rent for the space used to generate those sales will not change. This is because building rent is based on the value of building, which is not directly affected by changes in sales. Other examples of fixed costs include property taxes, managers' salaries, and business licenses. Pharmacies frequently have high fixed costs. Most pharmacies have to pay rent for a building, depreciation on invested assets like technology, manager pharmacist salaries, and other fixed costs not associated with changes in sales.

Pharmacist salaries are often fixed because state laws require a pharmacist to be present whenever prescription services are provided. In other cases, pharmacist time is dedicated to specific programs and services. A community pharmacy might hire a new pharmacist specifically to implement and operate a warfarin monitoring service and agree to pay her $100,000 per year regardless of the volume of warfarin monitoring services provided. In this case, the pharmacist's salary would be a fixed cost.

Variable costs rise in direct proportion to increases in volume of services and products provided. Sometimes an offering is structured to include significant variable costs. For example, a pharmacist who implements a smoking cessation clinic in a pharmacy might be reluctant to hire an additional pharmacist until he sees the demand for the service. Instead, he might pay one of the pharmacists involved in dispensing services to work additional hours to operate the smoking cessation service. In this situation, as the volume of services provided increases, so does the number of hours the pharmacist works. Since the service-related salary expense grows proportionately, salary expense for the service is a variable cost.

Direct and Indirect Costs

Another way of categorizing costs is as direct and indirect. *Direct costs* are those that are directly caused by or result from providing the service. Direct costs of providing a smoking cessation service include pharmacists' time spent counseling and educating patients, patient education materials, and the cost of any products (such as nicotine gum) used to assist patients in quitting. Direct costs may also be thought of as those costs that the pharmacy would not incur if it did not provide the service. If the pharmacy did not dispense prescriptions, it would not incur the costs of prescription containers or pharmacy licenses.

Indirect costs are those that are not directly caused by or do not directly result from providing the service. They are costs that the pharmacy would incur even if it did not provide the service in question. Examples include rent, utilities, and the manager's salary. These costs are shared costs or joint costs, in the sense that they are necessary for the sale of all the pharmacy's products and services. If the pharmacy did not provide smoking cessation services, it would continue to incur indirect costs.

There are excellent sources that describe how pharmacists can calculate the costs of their services.[4,5,6] Readers are directed to the references at the end of the chapter for details.

Step 3. Estimate Demand

Demand refers to the quantity of a product or service that consumers will buy at a given price. Demand for pharmacist services must be determined from the consumer's point of view. It is affected by consumer need, a consumer's perception of the pharmacist and pharmacy, perceptions of price and value, and availability of competing services.

Demand is affected by price. Classical economics states that as the price of a product or service rises, the quantity demanded by consumers typically falls. The extent to which the quantity demanded changes in response to price is known as the *price elasticity of demand*. It is a measure of how sensitive consumers are to different price levels. Different products and services have different levels of elasticity or price sensitivity. Knowing how sensitive consumers are to prices for a service—that is, knowing the demand for a service—is critical to setting an appropriate price.

Dolan[22] and Nagle and Holden[23] suggest that managers use the following guidelines to estimate consumers' price sensitivity for a specific product or service.

1. The consumer's sensitivity to price increases as the price of the product or service becomes a greater part of the total cost of therapy. The total cost of treating coughs and colds is low, so consumers are quite sensitive to the price of pharmacist counseling for cough and cold products. A high price for this service will probably result in little or no demand. The total treatment costs of asthma, on the other hand, are quite high. They include expensive drug therapy, frequent physician monitoring, trips to the emergency room, and hospitalizations. Compared with the total costs of treating asthma, the costs of asthma-related counseling provided by pharmacists are small. Therefore, consumers are likely to be less sensitive to the price of asthma counseling services.

2. Consumers' sensitivity to price is higher when they can compare prices and they perceive that there is little difference between competing products and services. The ability to compare prices depends on a consumer's perceived (not necessarily actual) competence to judge differences in quality and how convenient it is for them to do so. Nonprescription drugs, for example, are easy to compare. Neatly arrayed on a pharmacy shelf or online website, consumers can choose a product based upon recognition of a brand, recommendation from a pharmacist or friend, or previous experience. If they have no brand preference, they may be very price sensitive. The services of a surgeon, on the other hand, are not standardized. The quality of surgical services is difficult to assess and there is little good information available to permit price shopping. Plus, a bad decision could have severe consequences. Therefore, price sensitivity for surgical services is typically very low.

3. Consumers' price sensitivity increases as switching costs increase. Switching costs are the costs—both monetary and nonmonetary—that consumers incur when they change their source of supply for a product or service. If a particular pharmacy is much more convenient for consumers, then they may incur significant time costs in switching their purchases to another pharmacy. If patients have a warm personal and professional relationship with the pharmacist at that pharmacy, they may be less likely to respond to $25 coupons that encourage the transfer of prescriptions to a new pharmacy. If a PBM charges high copayments for medications received from pharmacies outside of the PBM's network, patients will be discouraged from trying new pharmacies.

Price as a Signal of Quality

There is a big exception to the rule that higher prices reduce demand for marketed products and services. This exception occurs when consumers use price as an indicator of quality. Price is used to indicate quality when objective measures of quality are not available. This is common in health care, which is more difficult to judge than typical consumer products.

Consumers often assume that higher-priced services are of higher quality. Consequently, pharmacists should think twice before pricing their services too low. Low prices may signal to patients that pharmacist services are trivial and cannot be justified with higher prices.

Nonmonetary Costs

Pharmacists should consider nonmonetary costs when estimating demand for their services. For instance, the cost of visiting a pharmacy includes not just what is paid for purchased merchandise. Patients also incur time costs for traveling to and waiting for pharmacy services to be delivered, plus search costs in trying to find the products and services they need. They incur psychic costs by worrying about whether their medicines will help or harm them. In many cases, these nonmonetary costs may mean more to consumers than monetary costs. Indeed, many pharmacists have difficulty enrolling patients in "free" medication therapy management (MTM) programs, because free does not mean "without cost".

Step 4. Set a Price

Based upon the price objective and estimates of cost and demand, a price can be set. Pharmacists should test price perceptions with customers and be willing to adjust prices based upon those perceptions. One rule of thumb is to err on the side of pricing a service too high rather than too low because it is easier to lower a price than raise it. Lowering a price can be promoted as offering a bargain, but a price increase cannot be promoted at all. And price increases will be looked at as a negative, even if the consumer is still willing to pay it. Consider how irritated people become when public utilities and cable companies announce price increases.

Step 5. Change the Price as Needed

Ideally, it would be nice if pharmacists could set their prices and forget about them. In real life, however, pricing strategies are situational and situations change. A new pharmacy that wants to rapidly build sales volume may offer low prices to attract business. But as business increases, price changes will be needed to increase the revenue needed to run the pharmacy.

Pharmacists should adjust prices based upon revenue targets for the overall portfolio (not just the individual product or service) and customer responses to what is offered. Some pricing might be dynamic, changing from week to week while other prices may be consistent over time. This occurs with some drug prices which change frequently. The end goal, however, is always to generate sufficient revenue to profitably stay in business.

NEW PAYMENT MODELS FOR PHARMACIST SERVICES

Up to this point, all discussions of pricing have revolved around fee-for-service models where each unit of service provided by a pharmacist is compensated for with the payment of a fee. Health care reform is driving new payment models for pharmacists and other health care providers. These include the following models:[24]

- Pay for Coordination - In this model, pharmacists are paid for specified care coordination services to providers. For example, pharmacists who contract with medical homes (i.e., health systems providing and coordinating primary care) may receive a monthly payment to coordinate the delivery of pharmaceutical care as patients transition from hospitals to community care.

- Pay for Performance - Pay for performance (P4P) is defined as a payment or bonus for achieving some specified performance goal. P4P is common in service contracts between pharmacies and health care insurers. In the past, performance was measured using non-clinical measures such as patient satisfaction scores and generic substitution rates. Now, clinical measures are being used in P4P including patient rates of medication adherence and appropriate medication use in special populations like persons with diabetes, asthma, and cardiovascular disease. The Centers for Medicare & Medicaid Services (CMS) uses the Medicare Star ratings system to reward high-quality pharmacy providers with bonuses and rebates.

- Episode or Bundled Payments - This model uses single payments for a group of services. These services might be related to a treatment or condition and may involve multiple providers in multiple settings. Pharmacies contract to receive all or a portion of the bundled payment to cover their role in treating the condition.

Most new payment models for pharmacist services use business-to-business (B2B) models instead of business-to-consumer (B2C) models of payment. B2B models occur when both the provider and customer are businesses. Examples of B2B models include pharmacies that enter into agreements with PBMs or local pharmacies that contract with nearby hospitals.

B2B pricing differs from B2C pricing because B2B purchases are typically much larger. Rather than transactions covering the needs of one patient, service contracts between businesses may cover the needs of thousands of people. B2B purchases are also more complex. Numerous individuals may be involved in contracting, managing, and monitoring the purchase agreement. Pharmacists may need to interact with people with various roles including initiating, influencing, deciding, approving, and completing the purchase. Because there are so many people involved, most businesses have standardized processes which make the final choice more likely to be based on objective criteria (e.g., return on investment) than what might be seen with B2C. Consumers are prone to being influenced by subjective preferences and emotion, while businesses tend to be evidence-based. Therefore, succeeding under new payment models requires knowing what is important to key organizational decision makers and using that information to craft a strong business case for the value of pharmacist services.

CONCLUSION

Pricing pharmacist services is a key activity to sustainably serving the needs of patients. Successful pricing requires understanding and thoughtfully considering a broad range of variables including the pharmacy's mission and objectives, costs of providing services and merchandise, demand for what is being offered, perspectives of decision makers, details about the market where services are provided, and customer psychology. Pharmacies that get pricing right can thrive. Those that do not will have trouble staying in business.

Reference List

(1) Schafermeyer KW, Schondelmeyer SW, Thomsas III J, Proctor KA. An analysis of the cost of dispensing third-party prescriptions in chain pharmacies. J Res Pharm Econ 1992;4(3):3-23.

(2) Grant Thornton LLP. National study to determine the cost of dispensing prescriptions in community retail pharmacies. Washington, DC: The Coalition for Community Pharmacy Action 2007.

(3) Carroll NV, Brusilovsky I, York B, Oscar R. Comparison of costs of community and mail service pharmacy. JAPHA-WASHINGTON- 2005;45(3):336.

(4) Carroll NV, Rupp MT, Holdford DA. Analysis of costs to dispense prescriptions in independently owned, closed-door long-term care pharmacies. J Manag Care Pharm 2014;20(3):291-300.

(5) Carroll N. Financial Management for Pharmacists: A Decision-Making Approach. Philadelphia: Lea & Febiger; 1991.

(6) Carroll N. Costs of dispensing private-pay and third-party prescriptions in independent pharmacies. Journal of Pharmaceutical Economics 1991;3:3-16.

(7) Rupp MT. Analyzing the costs to deliver medication therapy management services. J Am Pharm Assoc (2003) 2011;51(3):e19-e26.

(8) Rupp MT. Strategies for reimbursement. American Pharmacy NS32[Apr], 79-86. 1992.

(9) Brooks C. 6 Kinds of Deal Seekers and What They Mean to Your Business. 1-9-2014. Business News Daily. 2-7-2015.

(10) Porter ME. The five competitive forces that shape strategy. Harv Bus Rev 2008;86(1):78-93, 137.

(11) Pujol N. Freemium: attributes of an emerging business model. Available at SSRN 1718663 2010.

(12) Sussex J, Towse A, Devlin N. Operationalizing value-based pricing of medicines : a taxonomy of approaches. Pharmacoeconomics 2013;31(1):1-10.

(13) Raftery J. Value based pricing: can it work? BMJ 2013;347:f5941.

(14) Persson U, Svensson J, Pettersson B. A new reimbursement system for innovative pharmaceuticals combining value-based and free market pricing. Appl Health Econ Health Policy 2012;10(4):217-225.

(15) Farley JF, Wansink D, Lindquist JH, Parker JC, Maciejewski ML. Medication adherence changes following value-based insurance design. Am J Manag Care 2012;18(5):265-274.

(16) Choudhry NK, Fischer MA, Smith BF et al. Five features of value-based insurance design plans were associated with higher rates of medication adherence. Health Aff (Millwood) 2014;33(3):493-501.

(17) Wertz D, Hou L, DeVries A et al. Clinical and economic outcomes of the Cincinnati Pharmacy Coaching Program for diabetes and hypertension. Manag Care 2012;21(3):44-54.

(18) Porter ME. A strategy for health care reform--toward a value-based system. N Engl J Med 2009;361(2):109-112.

(19) Porter ME. Value-based health care delivery. Ann Surg 2008;248(4):503-509.

(20) Hamilton R, Chernev A. Low Prices Are Just the Beginning: Price Image in Retail Management. Journal of Marketing 2013;77(6):1-20.

(21) Bennett MS, Blank D, Bopp J, James JA, Osterhaus MC. Strategies to improve compensation for pharmaceutical care services. J Am Pharm Assoc (Wash) 2000;40(6):747-755.

(22) Dolan RJ. How do you know when the price is right? Long Range Planning 1995;28(6):125.

(23) Nagle TT, Holden RK. The Strategy and Tactics of Pricing: A Guide to ProfitableDecision Making. 3rd ed. Upper Saddle River,N.J.: Prentice Hall; 2002.

(24) Silversmith J. Five payment models: the pros, the cons, the potential. Minn Med 2011;94(2):45-48.

Chapter Questions

1. Discuss how offering medication therapy management services for free may reduce demand for those services.

2. List all of the costs to a community pharmacy that go into dispensing a single prescription for a newly prescribed antibiotic. List all of the nonmonetary costs to a patient that go into acquiring and taking a prescription for a newly prescribed antibiotic.

3. Compare and contrast price, compensation, reimbursement, charge, cost, and revenue. Which of these are largely outside of the control of pharmacists?

4. Who has more power in the pharmacy marketplace, pharmacists or the people who use pharmacist services? Suggest ways to increase the power of pharmacists.

5. Make a value-based argument for pharmacist services.

6. What are potential downsides to pharmacists relying on cost-plus pricing for their professional services?

7. Which new payment model described at the end of the chapter do you think will be most likely to stimulate the demand for medication therapy management? Why?

CHAPTER 14

MARKETING COMMUNICATION

Objectives

After studying this chapter, the reader should be able to

- o Discuss the purpose of promoting pharmacy products and pharmacist services
- o Explain barriers to effective marketing communication, using the communication model
- o Describe the information processing model
- o Use the information processing model to discuss the relative effectiveness of various communication media
- o List the six forms of promotion used to communicate marketing messages
- o Explain the advantages and disadvantages of each of these forms of promotion

Communication is the fuel that keeps the fire of your relationship burning, without it, your relationship goes cold.

— William Paisley

Communication is an essential component of the marketing mix. It is used to communicate with consumers the product being offered, the place it can be found, and the price offered. Without marketing communication, even a highly desirable, well-priced, and convenient product can fail.

Marketing communications are the tools used to communicate the promise made about a brand. Communications are more than just advertising. They comprise any contact between the marketer and customer that conveys a message to any of the five senses. This not only includes visual and audible messages, but smells, tastes, and textures.

Effective communications establish a clear image of the brand in the mind of the customers. It involves asking, "What value am I providing to my customers? How can I communicate that value in a way that is meaningful, clear, and memorable?"

To answer this question, the marketer needs to have a fundamental understanding of the targeted audience. This understanding is based upon observations of audience behaviors and conversations about needs and preferences. Like with any communication, marketing communications requires listening and watching. Marketing communications are also two way, with the customer responding to the communications verbally (e.g., conversation between a pharmacist and a patient), in writing (e.g., online evaluations) or through actions (e.g., purchases). This chapter discusses the psychology of marketing communications and the variety of ways of communicating.

MARKETING IN ACTION

Walgreens 'Find A Pharmacist' Online Directory

Walgreens launched an integrated marketing campaign back by televisions advertisements to promote its online "Find A Pharmacist" directory in 2012. Based upon Walgreens research that found that, in addition to location, consumers choose pharmacies based on a pharmacist's training and areas of expertise. Nearly 70% of respondents reported that they would be willing to switch pharmacies based upon the pharmacist serving them.

Patients can go onto the Walgreens website, click on the "Find A Pharmacist" tab, type in your location, and find pharmacists near you with specialties in medication adherence, immunizations, diabetes management, children's health, wellness education, medication side effects, and HIV care.

The "find a pharmacist" program permits consumers to make appointments with pharmacies if they have specific needs. They can ask the pharmacy when specific individuals are available to speak with them.

They can also use the directory to find out which local pharmacists can speak their language. If not, pharmacists can use the website to get in touch with one of the chain's 28,000 pharmacists, who speak a total of 16 languages, to translate for the customer in the store.

The online directory is available on mobile devices, and is integrated with other Walgreen's technology like the "refill by scan" feature, which allows consumers to scan bar codes on pill bottles and send in refill requests. The mobile device provides access to a "pill reminder" app and "Transfer by Scan" app too. Well filled, Walgreens sends refill reminder and "prescription-ready" text alerts to customers.

Source: Walgreens.com

PURPOSE OF MARKETING COMMUNICATIONS

Marketing communications consist of a range of media designed to:

INFORM ("Prescription refills now on the Internet!" "Immunizations will be offered from 10 am to 12 noon on Saturday"),

PERSUADE ("Our prices can't be beat!" "Our employees care about you"),

REMIND ("Don't forget! We're still America's most trusted" "Have you had your blood pressure checked recently?"), and/or

INFLUENCE BEHAVIORS ("Get a $25 reward coupon when you switch prescriptions." "'Like us' on Facebook").

Every word and action of pharmacists sends a message to the public. They communicate something about the image and professionalism of the pharmacist, the pharmacist's employer, and the profession. Communicating a desirable image about pharmacists and their value requires continual effort and conscious attention to the pharmacy brand.

It is frequently difficult to distinguish from marketing communications from pharmacist services because they both communicate messages and serve the needs of customers. When pharmacists serve patients, they also communicate an image about their professionalism and quality of services. When communicating with marketing media, they help patients by informing and reminding them about options and persuading them about which options can best meet patient needs. It is best to see marketing communications as being different but overlapping with pharmacist services. Both can serve and influence the pharmacy brand.

BRANDS

A primary purpose of marketing communications is to build and strengthen brands. A *brand* is a name, term, sign, symbol, design, or some combination of these that is intended to identify the goods and services of one seller or group of sellers and to differentiate them from those of competitors.[1] Promotional communications try to get people to attach some symbolic meaning to a brand. People associate the word Tylenol with quality, value, and relief. Google, Coke, and BMW are all associated with certain qualities in the minds of customers. Consumers who have positive perceptions of a brand are more likely to purchase or use that brand.

Walgreens, CVS, Rite Aid, Target, Kroger, and Wal-Mart are common brands in pharmacy. Each is associated with a level of satisfaction, quality, and value in the mind of customers. Brands evoke responses that can range from hate to no opinion to fanatic loyalty. It is the marketer's goal to establish and enhance positive images for brands in the minds of customers.

The word *pharmacist* is a powerful brand in the minds of many customers. It may suggest images of trust, reliability, professionalism, and competence. For other people, however, it may bring to mind the image of pill counter or, almost as bad, it may evoke no image at all.

Individual pharmacists have their own brands: their names. Each pharmacist's name is associated with an image in the minds of those who interact with him or her. Think of a pharmacist you know who has a good reputation. What words come to mind when you think of that person? It is likely that your image of the pharmacist was the result of hard work on the part of that individual. Successful pharmacists take great care in developing and maintaining the image associated with their name.

Brand Awareness

Brand awareness is the strength of a brand's presence in a consumer's mind.[1] It is the extent to which consumers (1) recognize a brand when they see it (i.e., brand recognition) and (2) recall it when asked to consider the product category (i.e., brand recall).

Brand recognition comes from any exposure to the brand through promotional communications, service experiences, or recommendations from friends. Brand recognition means simply that when given a list of brands, consumers say they have heard of the brand. It is a weak measure of awareness.

Recognition is important because people are more positive toward familiar things.[1] For instance, most people would choose a food they have tasted over foods they have never tasted. If food looks different from food we have tried in the past, we resist trying it. It often takes marketing promotions or recommendations from friends and family members to get us to try a new food.

Brand recall means that consumers think of the brand when asked to list brands in a product category. It is a stronger measure of awareness than brand recognition. The percentage of people who answer "pharmacist" when asked, "Who is the drug expert among health care professionals?" is a measure of brand recall.

Brands that are quickly recalled are more likely to be considered in consumer choices.[1] In addition to recall of products and services, recall of individual people can be important. Mary Jones, the pharmacist, has a much better chance of being considered for a promotion if her name comes to mind when her bosses are discussing personnel matters. In other words, Mary cannot be considered if her name never comes up.

Brand Image

Brand image, also called brand meaning, refers to the dominant perception of a brand in consumers' minds.[1] It is the image that immediately comes to mind upon hearing a name such as Starbucks, McDonald's, Wal-Mart, or Microsoft. Brand image can be positive, neutral, or negative.

Brand image is determined by the types and quality of associations made in the minds of consumers. Associations can be made through sounds (e.g., musical jingles), visual images (e.g., logos), and words (e.g., slogans). Ideally, brand associations should be favorable to the brand and of sufficient strength and uniqueness to be recognized and recalled. Brand image comes from a variety of sources:

- Customer experience. Every contact with a branded object helps shape its image. For a pharmacy, image is shaped by the look of the parking lot, window signs, interior store appearance, and interactions with pharmacy personnel. For a pharmacist, image is shaped by general appearance, tone of voice, body language, and many other factors.

- Promotional communications. Television, webpages, signage, and newspaper advertising present images of pharmacies and pharmacists. Image comes from the portrayal of pharmacists and pharmaceuticals in promotional messages.

- External information sources. These include word-of-mouth recommendations from friends and family and publicity in the general press.

Brand Equity

Branding provides value to a product. Consider branded laundry detergents. There is little actual difference between most laundry detergent brands, although their prices can vary considerably. The difference in price comes primarily from the brand image established through positioning. That difference in price is brand equity—the added value that a brand gives to a product or service.[1]

Brand equity is formed from a customer's awareness and perceived image of the brand.[1] Each element of the marketing mix helps influence perceptions of the brand and brand equity. When a pharmacy gives away professional services to patients or promotes low prescription drug prices, that affects the image of professional services. To protect the equity of the brand, pharmacists must carefully consider how marketing actions affect brand perceptions.

Although some critics might say that brands do nothing but add extra cost for the consumer, the consumer can benefit from brands. Brands can simplify the consumer's search for a product. The consumer simply looks for the trusted brand and makes the purchase. A good brand image can also reduce the buyer's perceived risk of making a bad decision. For instance, patients with serious health conditions tend to seek out physicians with the best reputation. Although other physicians may be equally good, the physician with the best reputation is the one most in demand. The greater the risk, the more important branding becomes in making a choice.

Marketers measure brand equity in two ways. The first is to assess consumer perceptions of the brand through studies of reputation or image. A strong reputation can help differentiate a seller's products and services from those of competitors. The second way to measure brand equity is to calculate the financial value added to a product as a result of increased sales and profits. Strong brands permit sellers to charge higher prices and derive greater profits.

Patients' image of pharmacies and individual pharmacists has a substantial influence on their loyalty, buying habits, and willingness to participate in therapy. Pharmacists and pharmacies that are able to project and maintain a positive brand image in the minds of customers are more likely to achieve success both professionally and financially.

THE COMMUNICATION PROCESS

To understand marketing communication, it is important to understand how consumers process the massive amount of information to which they are exposed. This includes how messages are sent, received, processed, and stored in memory. Familiarity with some simple models can help pharmacists maximize the effectiveness of their messages.

Whatever the message, all communications follow a common process (Figure 14-1). A sender (the marketer) has a message for a receiver (the consumer). The sender of the message must encode the message in words or images. The message (e.g., "Buy our product") may be in pictures, written words, spoken words, sounds, or symbols. The encoded message must be transmitted through some medium, such as television, radio, magazines, billboards, the Internet, or conversation. That message, under the right conditions, is then received and decoded (i.e., interpreted) by the receiver. Decoding of the message is influenced by factors such as the consumer's attention, attitudes, knowledge, and biases. In some cases the message received will prompt the receiver to act (e.g., buy the product). In many other cases the message is not acted on immediately and is either stored in memory for access at a later date or forgotten. All messages are transmitted in an environment full of the noise from thousands of other messages.

Many things can go wrong in the path represented by the communication process. The message may be poorly conceptualized, vague, or confusing. The desired receiver may miss the message, hear or see it incorrectly, interpret it wrong, or remember it inaccurately. With mass media (e.g., television or radio) communications, the problems are multiplied. A single message is sent to thousands or millions of receivers whose levels of sophistication, accessibility, and motivation are different, resulting in numerous interpretations of the same message. The message "Eat healthy food" can be perceived differently by people of diverse backgrounds and circumstances.

Marketing communication is complicated by the fact that we live in an age of constant distractions. People spend less time processing messages than they did in the past. The ever-increasing amount of information to which people are exposed has forced them to deal with information superficially.

Multitasking is common; people simultaneously watch TV, talk on the phone, surf the Web, and juggle other activities. Consumers are likely to skim promotional messages, gather bits and pieces of data, and incorporate the data into some understanding that may be broad but not deep. To successfully compete for the consumer's attention, marketing messages about products and services must be available, clear, consistent, and coherent.

This is why marketers often use segmentation to develop unique promotional plans for different target populations. The goal is to find a promotional message and medium appropriate for each target market. Each market segment should receive a message geared to its level of interest, knowledge, and attention. Table 14-1 illustrates how pharmaceutical salespeople modify their messaging to different categories of physicians to be most effective in influence prescribing habits.

Figure 14-1 The Communication Process

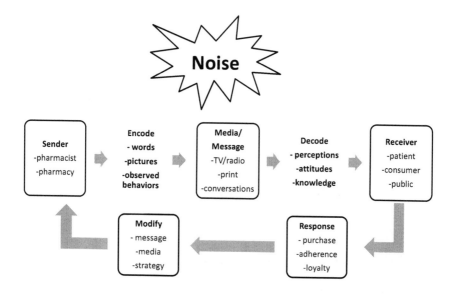

THE INFORMATION PROCESSING MODEL

Promotional communications face stiff competition for consumers' attention. No one really knows the real number of commercial messages the average person is exposed to daily, but it is in the hundreds, if not thousands. Of those, only a fraction are consciously noticed, and only a handful of the noticed messages provoke some form of reaction. The difficulty in getting consumers' attention causes some marketers to do whatever it takes to be noticed, including placing their messages on almost anything (e.g., urinals, people's bodies, food products), anywhere (e.g., in movies and television shows, schools and public buildings).

Even when consumers do notice a promotional message, it may not be perceived in the way the marketer intended. In many cases, consumers distort the message so that they hear what they want to hear. In other cases, consumers lack the time, knowledge, or ability to interpret the message correctly.

Table 14-1 Approaches for communicating with different physician market segments

Physician Segment	Messaging Approach
Friendly and Outgoing	All messages are framed as a gesture of friendship. "I give them free samples not because it's my job, but because I like them so much. I provide office lunches because visiting them is such a pleasant relief from all the other docs."
Aloof and Skeptical	Journal articles are provided to counter doctors' concerns about drug shortcomings. "I play dumb and have the doc explain to me the significance of my article."
Mercenary	Messages are transactional, "If you prescribe drug x, I will do these nice things for you."
High-prescribers	Strong personal connections are made to make the salesperson stand out from other salespeople.
Prefers a Competing Drug	The key is to understand why the physician is using the competitor and frame messages to counter these preferences.
Acquiescent Docs	These physicians avoid conflict and simply agree to requests. Get the physician to agree and move on to the next one.
No-see/ No-time (hard-to-see docs)	If the physician is unavailable, spend time and money on office staff and nurses. They can help the salesperson influence the busy doctor.
Thought Leaders	Groom friendly thought leaders to speak at meetings and paid dinners. Encourage further speaking engagements if they show loyalty toward company products.

Source: Reference[2]

Pharmacists who wish to enhance the effectiveness of their promotional communications need to understand how consumers process information—how they receive it, interpret it, and store it in personal memory. The information processing model in Figure 11-2 describes consumer decision-making as similar to a funnel where each step in the process allows fewer and fewer messages through.

Between the sender sending a message and the receiver's response are five steps:

1. *Exposure.* The first step in marketing communication is to expose the receiver to the message. This requires selecting a medium that will get the message to the target receiver.

2. *Attention.* Next, the message must capture the attention of the receiver. The medium should be able to provide the message in a way that appeals to the interest of the receiver and can compete with the thousands of other messages people are exposed to daily.

3. *Comprehension.* Attention then needs to lead to comprehension of the intended message. There are many ways to misunderstand a message. Comprehension depends, in part, on the receiver's motivation, knowledge, and biases. It is best for the message to be simple, vivid, and clear.

4. *Acceptance.* Messages that are clearly communicated and comprehended are not necessarily accepted. Many smokers clearly understand antismoking messages but do not accept them.

5. *Retention.* Even messages that are accepted are often forgotten. Messages need to be memorable. Humor or imagery can be used to establish the message in the receiver's mind. Repetition can also reinforce the image in memory.

In the information processing model, messages must progress through several stages before they can lead to a desired action. Only messages that reach the consumer, grab his or her attention, are understood, are accepted, and remembered will be effective. Failure at any stage of the model means ultimate failure of the communication.

Figure 14-2 The information processing model

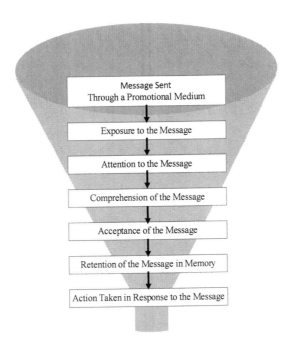

Pharmacists can use this information processing model to evaluate the effectiveness of different messages in influencing the actions of customer groups. For example, the effectiveness of the following communication methods for influencing physician prescribing practices could be evaluated:

o   Educational brochures directed to "Occupant,"

o   Personalized letters to individual physicians to accompany printed educational materials,

o   Patient-specific lists of prescribed medications,

o   Continuing-education (CE) programs during lunch at a physician's office, and

o   Face-to-face conversations with clinical pharmacists or other physicians.

Each of these communication forms has advantages and disadvantages. Educational brochures and personalized letters are inexpensive to produce and mail but are largely ineffective in influencing physician behavior.[3, 4] The effectiveness of printed materials is low because physicians often do not read them. Materials may be screened by a secretary or thrown out unopened by the physician. Even when they are read, printed materials may be only superficially scanned for relevant information. Thus, printed messages frequently fail in the exposure or attention step of the information processing model. Personalizing the message with the physician's name or specific patient prescribing information may increase attention somewhat, but comprehension, acceptance, and retention of printed information usually are still low, so the message has relatively little impact on prescribing behavior.[3, 4]

Oral communication of messages through CE programs might be expected to achieve greater levels of attention and comprehension than print media. CE programs tend to attract people who are interested in the subject matter and more receptive to the messages being communicated. However, interaction between the speaker and the audience often is low, and drifting audience attention may diminish the acceptance and retention of the message. The effectiveness of CE programs in influencing physician prescribing is small at best.[3]

The most effective form of communication for influencing physician prescribing is face-to-face conversation. This is commonly referred to as *academic detailing* or *counterdetailing*.[4, 5] The term academic detailing originated with prescribing interventions at teaching institutions. The term counterdetailing is used because these interventions were initially designed to counteract information provided to physicians by pharmaceutical sales personnel (called detailers). Face-to-face communication, unlike print material, cannot easily be ignored. Comprehension and acceptance are enhanced because the message can be tailored to the interests and understanding of the physician. Retention of the message is reinforced because the presentation is more interactive.

Electronic systems offer further opportunity to influence prescribing. They enable pharmacists and others to communicate with physicians at the point of prescribing. Physicians can be informed, persuaded, and reminded through targeted messages, personalized educational interventions, updates, and electronic consultations. Relevant information can be provided when it is needed, in a way that is hard to ignore. Communications can be individualized to be more engaging and acceptable to physicians and thus more likely to be understood and acted upon.

PROMOTIONAL METHODS

In communicating their messages to targeted audiences, marketers use various methods of promotion that can be divided into two categories: *marketer controlled* and *marketer influenced* (Figure 11-3). In marketer-controlled methods, the message, medium, and delivery are directly managed through monetary payment. Advertising, personal selling, direct marketing, and sales promotions are marketer controlled; compensation is paid to the person or entity that delivers the message (e.g., the salesperson or advertising firm). In contrast, promotional methods that are marketer influenced do not involve quid pro quo compensation from the marketer to the entity delivering the message. Instead, marketers indirectly influence the messages through what are called *third-party techniques*. The strategies employed here separate the message from the self-interested messenger (i.e., the marketer);[6] they include public relations and word-of-mouth ("buzz") communications.

MARKETER-CONTROLLED METHODS

Advertising, personal selling, direct marketing, and sales promotions differ in how they communicate marketing messages. Differences include the number of people likely to be exposed to the message (this is termed *reach*), cost per person reached, and level of impact on consumer behavior. The advantages and disadvantages of each method are described in the following sections.

> Half the money I spend on advertising is wasted; the trouble is I don't know which half.
>
> —John Wanamaker, Marketing Pioneer

Advertising

Advertising is any paid, nonpersonal presentation promoting ideas, goods, or services.[7] It includes print messages (e.g., in newspapers, magazines, newsletters, outdoor ads, and Yellow Pages), broadcast messages (e.g., television, radio, podcasting), and Internet advertising (e.g., Web site banners).

Advertising in large newspapers or on radio or television is likely to be out of the financial reach of small pharmacy operations. However, small businesses can take advantage of a variety of low-priced, local advertising media, such as telephone Yellow Pages advertisements, business directory listings, fliers posted on bulletin boards in community buildings and businesses, advertisements in programs of community and high school theater groups, and penny-saver newspaper advertisements.

In addition to being less expensive, advertisements in local media may be perceived as more personal than those in major media such as television and magazines. Another advantage is that consumers tend to search local media for solutions to their problems. They are more likely to look at bulletin boards or in Internet Yellow Pages to find local businesses to serve their needs.

Figure 14-3 Promotional Methods

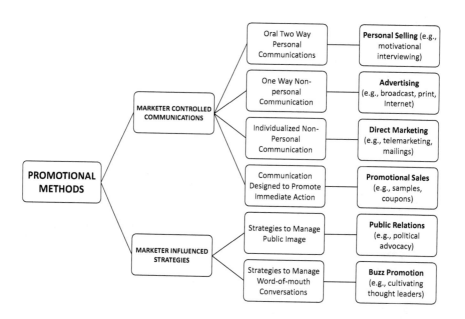

Personal Selling

Personal selling is any oral presentation to customers as individuals or groups.[7] As a promotional method, it differs from advertising because it permits immediate two-way communication. It is also the one promotional method engaged in by every pharmacist,[8] with varying levels of success. Personal selling activities in pharmacy include patient counseling, telephoning physicians to get them to change a patient's therapy, giving hospital in-service presentations for nurses, participating in hospital grand rounds, having brown bag meetings, and academic detailing.

Pharmacists may not like having their patient and professional interactions characterized as personal selling—as sales promotion instead of health promotion. This concern relates to the word "selling." A better word might be "consultation." Consultation is consistent with the concept of modern personal selling, which emphasizes long-term relationships that serve the customer and discourages short-sighted tactics to promote quick sales. Good personal selling helps customers use the product effectively, efficiently, and in a way that maximizes benefits over time—goals consistent with motivational interviewing and medication therapy management.

Direct Marketing

Direct marketing is individualized, nonpersonal communication.[7] It is individualized because it targets individual consumers, and it is nonpersonal because consumer contacts come from a database. Database marketing, direct mail, mail order, interactive technology, and computerized telemarketing are other terms used for this type of promotional communication.

The primary components of direct marketing are a customer database and a delivery medium (Figure 14-4). The database contains demographic information, purchasing habits, credit history, behavioral characteristics, and other information collected from a variety of sources, including Web sites, customer surveys, and loyalty card use. The more information the database contains, the more useful it is for identifying and targeting customers. The delivery vehicle is the medium used to contact database customers with a message or offer. Targeted customers might receive discount coupons, free samples, free or discounted services, or reminder messages.

Overuse and misuse of direct marketing has added to negative feelings toward the marketing profession.[9] Most complaints about marketers relate to the intrusive nature of direct marketing; they tend to focus on direct mail, telephone solicitation, or Internet spam. Consumers have learned to cope somewhat by screening or ignoring the messages. State and federal laws have also been passed to regulate direct marketers. The federal Health Insurance Portability and Accountability Act regulates how consumer health data can be collected and used. The Federal Trade Commission's National Do Not Call Registry allows consumers to bar telemarketers from calling them.

Sales Promotion

Sales promotion is any promotional communication used to promote a quick sale or action.[7] Examples include price deals, consumer coupons, contests and sweepstakes, refunds and rebates, premium offers, trade promotions, point-of-purchase displays at checkouts, in-store demonstrations, shows and exhibitions, stamps, and sample distribution.

Sales promotion is used to achieve short-term marketing objectives. It promotes immediate behavior, such as purchase of a product or participation in a service. Pharmacies use sales promotion to encourage the sale of merchandise and services. They may have senior citizen days, when all seniors receive a discount on purchases. Using coupons in weekly newspaper advertisements and mailed circulars is also common. Pharmacists frequently waive fees for certain services to reward loyal customers, or offer free initial consultations that encourage patients to sample clinical services. Although pharmacists may not recognize these fee waivers as sales promotion, they are, in effect, a price discount for services.

MARKETING IN ACTION

Customer Relationship Management at CVS

CVS analyzes purchasing data to develop programs to attract and retain customers. Their goal is to increase CVS pharmacy's share of wallet. Called customer relationship management (CRM), they use data from their millions cardholders enrolled in the ExtraCare® program to craft specific promotions. ExtraCare® customers in the program can earn ExtraBucks® at a rate of 2 percent on most in-store and online purchases and $1 for every two prescriptions purchased. These ExtraBucks® can be used in stores and when shopping online. Program customers receive e-mails and direct mailings with health and beauty tips, new product information, and discount coupons,

Information on ExtraCare® customer purchases can help identify opportunities for cross-promotions (i.e., or targeting customers of one product or service with a promotion for a related product) like sales promotions on toothbrushes for customers buying toothpaste.

ExtraCare® customers are also targeted with special promotions to increase their average spending per visit. For example, a $4 coupon might be offered to customers who normally spend $15 per visit for purchases of $25 or more.

ExtraCare® customers opt-in to the program and can opt-out whenever they want. This helps customers who want to protect their privacy or avoid the tailored messaging.

CRM programs like ExtraCare® account for over 20 percent of sales at drugstore chains. They can increase sales but lower gross margins by giving some of the profits back to customers in savings. The key to CRM success is to experiment with different messages and offers and use the results of those experiments to determine which promotions are most profitable.

Source: warrington.ufl.edu/centers/retailcenter/

Sales promotions can be aimed at either consumers or businesses. Those aimed at businesses are called *trade promotions.* They are used by manufacturers and others to encourage retail businesses to put extra effort into promoting certain targeted products. A manufacturer of a nonprescription medication or other product might offer a cash rebate if a certain sales volume of the product is achieved. Sales promotions can hurt pharmacist–patient relationships. Frequent use of discounts could tempt longtime patients to bounce from pharmacy to pharmacy.

Sales promotions can attract the least profitable customers. Pharmacy sales promotions are likely to attract patients who are more interested in getting discounts than in maintaining a long-term relationship with their pharmacist. These customers are often more costly than loyal customers. Discounts from sales promotions can be very expensive. Waiving patient co-payments or offering $25 off for switching a prescription can take a large bite out of a pharmacy's profits.

Sales promotions can be perceived as manipulative. They reward customers for jumping through hoops. This can irritate customers and is a major reason that some stores offer everyday low prices and minimize sales promotions.

MARKETER-INFLUENCED METHODS

Public relations and word-of-mouth marketing (commonly called "PR" and "WOM," respectively) are forms of promotion that are influenced, but not controlled, by marketers. Public relations is defined as the process of building a positive image in the minds of the public.[10] It is used to create a supportive climate in the community for your marketing initiatives. Word-of-mouth ("buzz") marketing stimulates discussion of products and services by potential customers.[11] While public relations promotes positive images, buzz marketing promotes positive conversation.

Public relations and buzz marketing are third-party techniques; they exert influence indirectly, through parties that are considered to be independent of marketers because they have no clear financial interest in the message. Third-party communications are perceived as more neutral and unbiased than paid forms of promotion such as advertising. This perception can increase attention to and acceptance of the message.

The major advantage of third-party communications—the independence of the communicators—is also a disadvantage. Third parties have no vested interest in conveying the message in the way the marketer desires, and they may distort, ignore, or contest the message. Negative images can be generated just as easily as positive ones. In fact, unfavorable news is likely to spread faster than good news.

Public Relations

Public relations encompasses a broad range of activities to build goodwill and a favorable image of a product or service in the eyes of the public.[10] Pharmacy's "publics," or stakeholders, range from the press to patients to funding agencies.

In the past, public relations was defined by marketers as any nonpaid attempt to get favorable coverage by the news media or to prevent negative coverage. Now, that definition is considered to describe a subset of public relations—publicity. The definition of public relations has been expanded to activities that include[10]

- Lobbying—advocating for a cause with legislatures and government agencies,
- Government relations—communicating with and educating legislatures and government agencies,
- Media relations—dealing with the media to seek publicity or stimulate interest in a cause,

- Publicity—communicating with the public through media (e.g., press releases, news conferences),
- Direct communications with constituents,
- Public appearances before groups (e.g., speeches, seminars), and
- Community relations—dealing with citizens and groups within an area.

Public relations promotes goodwill between marketers and the public. Goodwill toward the pharmacy profession is formed from positive images of and mental associations with pharmacists, pharmacy employees, and pharmacies. Public relations attempts to build positive images where they are absent, strengthen existing positive images, and repair any negative images that exist. The stronger and more positive the image communicated, the greater are the goodwill and consequent support for a cause.

Publicity is a key element of public relations. Pharmacists use publicity extensively to influence media coverage of the profession. Media coverage can be generated by

- Speaking to a community group about nonprescription medications,
- Participating in an "adopt-a-highway" program,
- Sponsoring a baseball team,
- Lobbying to expand the role of pharmacists,
- Demonstrating a new flavoring system to make drugs more acceptable to pediatric patients,
- Holding poison prevention programs,
- Sending National Pharmacy Week press releases,
- Offering free blood pressure screenings,
- Sponsoring public service announcements, and
- Writing letters to the editor about negative depiction of a pharmacist in the news.

Publicity events may cost money, but they are often less expensive than advertising and other forms of promotional communication. The primary cost results from the time and effort spent managing the message (which can be considerable).

The negative side of promotion through publicity is that, once in the hands of the media, the message can be ignored, de-emphasized, or distorted. Indeed, a television reporter can turn a pharmacist interview originally focused on how pharmacists reduce medication errors into a story about how pharmacists are not doing enough to reduce errors.

Word-of-Mouth Marketing

Word-of-mouth or buzz marketing encourages unpaid but influential individuals to generate conversation about ideas, products, or services.[11] Buzz has a connection to public relations; just as good public relations can cause buzz, buzz can cause good public relations. The primary difference is that buzz marketing focuses on promoting in-person discussion, while public relations emphasizes the development of goodwill.

Buzz spreads when extraordinary things are talked about. When people are exposed to a noteworthy idea or object, they want to tell others. The more remarkable or "sticky" the topic, the more likely it is to generate buzz. The value of buzz lies in its ability to encourage people to try new products, adopt fresh ideas, and use innovations.

MARKETING IN ACTION

"Monster Spray" Becomes a Viral Hit

A 6-year-old North Dakota girl had trouble sleeping at night knowing that there were monsters hiding in her bedroom. Employees at Barrett Pharmacy in Waterford City gave the 6-year-old a bottle of "Monster Spray" to spritz around her room at night. The special formula worked, and the girl was reported to be sleeping much better now.

The medicine has been used periodically over the years for young pharmacy customers and comes with its own prescription and instructions.

"Spray around the room at night before bed, repeat if necessary," the label reads.

A picture of the bottle was posted on Facebook and received 100 likes from friends. Then one of those "friends" shared the image and story with someone, who shared it with someone else and so on. Eventually, the story and image was picked up and reported on at an Evansville, Indiana radio station's Facebook page, drawing more than 245,000 likes and 71,000 shares. Then the image started appearing on Twitter, Pinterest, and other sites. The Imgur site recorded more than 720,000 views in three months.

Now, a web search of "monster spray" shows over 16 million results for news articles, images of various monster sprays for sale, and how-to Youtube videos.

Source: Reference[12]

SOCIAL MEDIA MARKETING

Social media marketing was not mentioned in previous editions of this book because it is a recent phenomenon. Things have changed quickly regarding social media and marketing. Old media like newspapers, radio, and television are diminishing in importance in communicating with customers. Now, social networks and media sharing sites are now essential in marketing communications.

Social media marketing is defined as the use of social media to serve the needs and wants of customers. It differs from traditional marketing because it works within a social media ecosystem.[13]

Although similar to traditional media in that marketers can broadcast one-way messages (i.e., podcast), engage in personal selling (e.g., instant messaging), direct market (e.g., opt-in to e-mail messages), promote action (e.g., electronic coupons), spread buzz (e.g., promote trending of web posts), and influence public relations (e.g., e-mail campaign), it differs by the speed, economy, and spread of messages.

In social media marketing, consumers and marketers interact with social media platforms like content sharing sites, blogs, social networking, and wikis to create, modify, share, and discuss Internet content.[14] Consumer engagement in this process is key to social media marketing.

Primary Forms of Social Media

The thousands of social media available to consumers fall into the following major categories.

Social networking sites - social networks that allow people to connect with each other and share comments and media (Facebook and Linkedin).

Bookmarking - Sites that allow users to save and organize online resources and links to popular websites (StumbleUpon).

Social news sites - these allow users to post news links to posted articles on the Internet. Users rate or vote on posts, and those with the highest ratings get most prominently displayed (Reddit).

Media sharing - websites that allow users to share media like photos and video. Sites typically offer the ability to create profiles and comment on uploaded media (YouTube).

Blogging and forums - sites that encourage users to have conversations through posts and blog comments. Conversations usually revolve around specific topics (WordPress).

Microblogging - these sites allow users to post short, written content or other media (Twitter).

Individuals engage in social media for a variety of reasons. There are seven functional things building blocks to the extent that they engage in social media[14]

1. **Share Identity** - extent to which users reveal their identities and information about themselves in a social media setting. Sharing identity is important in developing strong relationships between social media partners.[15]

2. **Establish Presence** - extent to which users can know if other users are accessible. Social media sites facilitate interactions in the virtual and real world by allowing users to know where others are located and what they are doing.

3. **Develop and Maintain Relationships** - extent to which users can connect with other users. These connections allow people to converse, share, meet up, or simply give a thumbs-up.

4. **Have Conversations** - extent to which users communicate with other users in a social media setting. The value of many social media sites comes from facilitating conversations among individuals and groups.

5. **Be Part of Groups** - extent to which users can form and interact with communities and subcommunities. These communities can be of any type (e.g., professional) or topic (e.g., greyhound rescue).

6. **Establish and Promote Reputations** - extent to which users can identify the standing of others, including themselves, in a social media setting. Reputation might be measured by the number of recommendations, likes, followers, or other reputational metrics.

7. **Sharing Things** - extent to which users exchange, distribute, and receive content. Sharing increases buzz through the internet and increases the impact of exchanges between people.

The degree to which marketers focus on some or all of these blocks helps determine the level and type of desired customer engagement with social media. By definition, social media is interactive, not passive. At minimum, it requires some form of connection with the media. At its highest level, it includes content creation and sharing with others. Figure 11-4 illustrates types of social media users.

Figure 14-4 Types of Social Media User

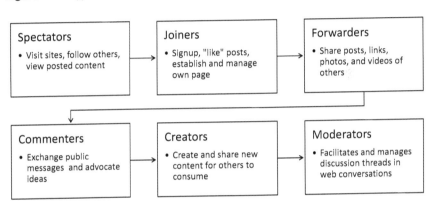

Pharmacists are using social media to serve and communicate with customers. They can help educate and influence large numbers of patients, while offering tailored messages to effectively target specific populations.[16] In addition, they can help promote public health by facilitating conversations, organizing groups of like-minded individuals, and share public health information.[16]

Pharmacists need to become familiar with how their customers engage with social media. Most of the media is easy to use and require minimal technical skills . The amount of time pharmacists need to invest depends on what they want to do. At minimum, pharmacists need to establish a web presence by have a Facebook page. Then it is important to maintain and update that with periodic updates.

Reference List

(1) Aaker D. Building Strong Brands. New York: The Free Press; 1996.

(2) Fugh-Berman A, Ahari S. Following the script: how drug reps make friends and influence doctors. PLoS Medicine 2007;4(4):e150.

(3) Smith WR. Evidence for the effectiveness of techniques to change physician behavior. Chest Journal 2000;118(2_suppl):8S-17S.

(4) Soumerai SB, Avorn J. Principles of educational outreach ('academic detailing') to improve clinical decision making. JAMA 1990;263(4):549-556.

(5) Avorn J, SB S. Improving drug-therapy decisions through educational outreach: A randomized controlled trial of academically based retailing. N Engl J Med 1983;308(24):1457-1463.

(6) Burton B, Rowell A. Unhealthy spin. BMJ: British Medical Journal 2003;326(7400):1205.

(7) Kotler P. Marketing Management: Analysis, Planning, and Control. 4th ed. Engelwood Cliffs, NJ: Prentice Hall; 1980.

(8)McDonough RP, Doucette WR. Using personal selling skills to promote pharmacy services. J Am Pharm Assoc (2003) 2003;43(3):363-372.

(9) Hackett R. How online pharmacy spammer organizations really work. Fortune Magazine . 11-21-2014. 2-3-2015.

(10) Pugliese TL. Public Relations for Pharmacists. Washington, DC: American Pharmacists Association; 2000.

(11) Holdford DA. Using buzz marketing to promote ideas, services, and products. Journal of the American Pharmacists Association: JAPhA 2003;44(3):387-395.

(12) Smart Retailing. One Monster Success. smartretailingrx com/marketing-promotions/one-monster-success/ 2014 April 11.

(13) Hanna R, Rohm A, Crittenden VL. We are all connected: The power of the social media ecosystem. Business horizons 2011;54(3):265-273.

(14) Kietzmann JH, Hermkens K, McCarthy IP, Silvestre BS. Social media? Get serious! Understanding the functional building blocks of social media. Business horizons 2011;54(3):241-251.

(15) Morgan RM, Hunt SD. The commitment-trust theory of relationship marketing. the journal of marketing 1994;20-38.

(16) Cain J, Romanelli F, Fox B. Pharmacy, social media, and health: Opportunity for impact. Journal of the American Pharmacists Association: JAPhA 2009;50(6):745-751.

Chapter Questions

1. Use the communication model in Figure 14-1 to describe why it is so hard for marketers to get their messages to consumers.

2. Use the information processing model in 14-2 to compare the relative effectiveness of a newspaper pharmacy advertisement, a television advertisement, a Facebook post, and personal selling by a pharmacist in getting a patient to take some action.

3. What are important things to consider when designing a marketing communication?

4. Discuss factors that go into a pharmacy's choice of a promotional medium.

5. Why might selling patient data to drug companies for direct marketing hurt the image of pharmacists?

CHAPTER 15

MARKETING COMMUNICATION STRATEGIES

Objectives

After studying this chapter, the reader should be able to

o List steps in developing a promotional plan
o Describe the purpose of positioning strategy statements and value propositions
o Develop positioning strategy statements and value propositions
o Delineate problems faced when crafting promotional messages
o Identify strategies to overcome problems with advertising pharmacy services

If you can't explain it to a six year old, you don't understand it yourself

—Albert Einstein

Marketing communications are a set of tools and strategies used to achieve an organization's mission. Like other elements of the marketing mix, they must be thoughtfully planned and implemented. Marketing messages must be crafted and delivered in a way that reaches targeted individuals, captures their attention, and is easily understood, accepted, and remembered. Messaging should convey a distinct, desired image of the pharmacy brand to targeted customers (e.g., friendly and professional).

Pharmacists must decide what to say and how to say it in words, images, and observed actions. Messages need to be organized and communicated in a way that distinguishes their services from competitors. Marketing communications must be integrated to coordinate multiple messages, media, channels, and propositions that are consistent and memorable. And all of this must to be done on a limited budget.

This chapter discusses strategies for effectively communicating with customers to achieve desired outcomes. It emphasizes strategies available to the average pharmacist who has little money to spend on marketing communications.

MARKETING IN ACTION

Rebranding Chemotherapy with an Assist from Superheroes

The nasty process of giving chemotherapy to children was made easier by a hospital in Brazil. Teaming up with Warner Bros., the cancer center created a story line in which superheroes undergo similar treatment with the children.

To raise the spirits of children, they were given the "Superformula", not chemotherapy. This superformula gave them the superpowers to vanquish their arch enemy, cancer. With the permission of Warner Bros. to use Justice League characters, child-size intravenous bags were given a makeover using covers that evoked characters like Batman and Wonder Woman.

The look of the children's ward was also changed with the game room now acting as the Hall of Justice and an entrance that reinforces the superhero theme.

Source: [1]

DEVELOPING AND IMPLEMENTING A COMMUNICATIONS PLAN

A communications plan is an element of the overall marketing plan that outlines how and what will be communicated to customers and others. Any plan must be founded on a clear understanding of the product, customers, competitors, price, and target market. Therefore, final details of the plan should only be crafted after all other elements of the business plan are decided. A promotional plan typically consists of the following steps:

1. Define the objective of the promotion,
2. Craft a message and means for delivering it,
3. Select an integrated communication mix,
4. Assess the effectiveness of the communications, and
5. Conduct a communications audit.

1. DEFINE THE OBJECTIVE

Communications objectives should originate from and complement the overall objectives established in the marketing plan, so that they will supplement and reinforce other elements of the marketing mix. Accordingly, if a pharmacist's professional image is a major part of the overall plan, then pricing, communications, pharmacy location, and all other elements of the marketing mix should reinforce this image of professionalism.

Promotional objectives typically revolve around a positioning strategy statement. The *positioning strategy statement* defines the product or services provided, target consumer, market, competition, and meaningful features of the product or business that differentiate it from competitors. The positioning statement may also describe the personality or image of the brand, which will be established and reinforced in all promotional communications. The following is an example of a positioning strategy statement that might be written for a community pharmacy:

Johnson's Apothecary provides professional pharmacist services, pharmacy products, and merchandise to consumers on the north side of the city and commuters in the northern suburbs. Johnson's Apothecary is a locally owned, family-run organization that takes care of people, not medical conditions. The owner and other pharmacists are well known and respected in the community. Two pharmacists are certified diabetes educators. The merchandise selection emphasizes health care over general merchandise. Personal service is paramount. Johnson's is also a meeting place for locals who want to chat with neighbors and friends.

Large pharmacy organizations may have more than one statement depending on what is being positioned (Figure 15-1). A pharmacy chain may have a broad positioning statement to convey their marketing message to customers, investors, and other key groups. A store within the chain may build upon the parent organization's messaging to position itself more precisely to the customers it serves and the local community. The store's positioning statement can be used to integrate the positioning of key products within the store, like a diabetes management program. Pharmacists who offer specific products to their customers, like professional services, must ensure that their positioning is consistent with the pharmacy in which it is provided and the corporation in which the pharmacist works.

All marketing communications should bolster the images promoted in the positioning statements. Sales promotions, advertising, and public relations events should be crafted with an eye toward their contribution to a consistent image. This will help ensure that the same message is repeated in multiple ways and media.

FIGURE 15-1 Levels of pharmacy positioning statements

Product – positioning a specific product like a diabetes management program in the minds of targeted customers

Pharmacy Store – positioning the pharmacy in the minds of the local community and customers

Pharmacy Chain – positioning the corporation in the minds of shareholders and the public

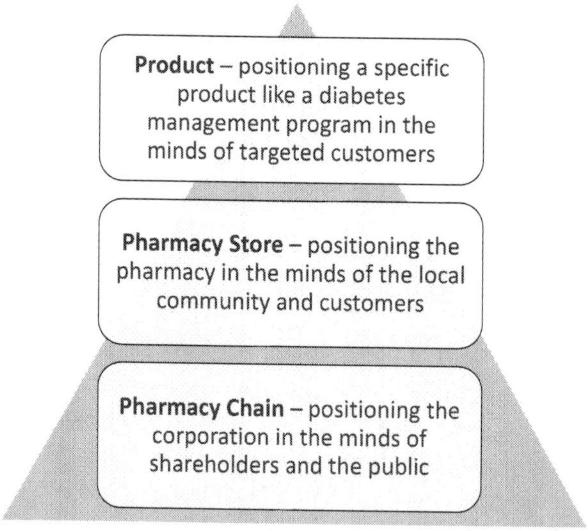

2. CRAFT A MESSAGE AND MEANS FOR DELIVERING IT

In Chapter 14, we learned from models of *The Communication Process* and *Information Processing* that there are a lot of ways for messages to fail. They can fail if the message is poorly conceptualized, vague, or confusing. The desired receiver may miss the message, hear or see it incorrectly, interpret it wrong, or remember it inaccurately. Messages that are clearly communicated and comprehended may not be accepted. Even if the message informs, persuades, and reminds effectively, it may not result in the intended action by the customer.

Crafting a message and means for delivering it requires marketers to answer 4 questions:

1. *What do I say (message content)?* How will my message appeal to my audience's self-interest, emotions, or moral viewpoints?
2. *How do I say what I want in words (message structure)?* Will the message be evenhanded or biased? How will the message be organized? Will the message take an emotional or cognitive approach?
3. *How do I say what I want in images (message format)?* What images or pictures will be used to get the message across? Will the medium used to communicate the message be able to convey the images in an effective way?
4. *Who should say it (message source)?* Will the source of the message be attractive and engaging enough to achieve high levels of attention and recall? Will the source convey the desired expertise and trustworthiness?

Value Proposition

The content of all promotional messages should revolve around some unique value proposition or "big idea." Value propositions are statements that summarize why a consumer should buy a product or use a service by a pharmacy or pharmacist. A value proposition is a promise of the value to be delivered to the customer or partner. It makes the case, either directly (e.g., "We are the best!") or subtly (e.g., "Isn't it time to try someone new?") for why someone should buy or use a product or service instead of a competing option.

The value proposition explains why a service solves a problem or makes things better for the customer. For example, a value proposition to a physician about a new medication adherence solution might say, "This service provides physicians with a comprehensive solution to the problem of patient medication nonadherence in one affordable package. The main features are..."

The value proposition is critical to crafting messages. To create a value proposition, pharmacists must be able to answer the following questions:

- Who is the *primary audience* for this value proposition? Different audiences may need different value propositions. A value proposition for a diabetes management clinic might vary for diabetics, the physicians treating those diabetics, an employer who is insuring diabetics, and a PBM who wants to control diabetic drug costs.
- *What is the problem (or problems) faced by your customers* for which you intend to offer a solution (e.g., non-adherence with medications, uncontrolled warfarin levels, lost productivity of employees due to health related problems)?
- *What are the main features* of the product or service to be provided (e.g., "The service consists of a five step process that...")?
- *How does it compare* with what is currently in the marketplace (e.g., "There are few programs designed for improving medication adherence in Richmond, and the ones which are available do not...")?
- *What evidence can you provide* to support your value proposition? Has this product or service been shown to work elsewhere (e.g., "A recent study published in the New England Journal of Medicine shows that this program...")? Is there a good logical argument to be made that your service will solve the problem(s)?

Evidence in support of value propositions are summarized in "proof points". A *proof point* is a statement or fact that provides undeniable evidence of a claim. Without proof points, claims of value sound like empty boasts or wishful thinking. Therefore, a pharmacy that claims, "We're your local medication therapy experts.", should follow up that statement with a proof point like, "All of our pharmacists are board certified." If it claims, "We're the best in town."; that claim should follow with something like, "Rated the best pharmacy in town for the last five years by Richmond Magazine."

There are many ways to craft value propositions. One way[2] consists of having three parts. The first part is a headline consisting of one short sentence describing the end-benefit of using a product. The headline may mention the product and/or the customer. The second part is a sub-headline or a short 2 to 3 sentence paragraph which explains what is offered, for whom, and why is it useful. The final part consists of approximately three bullet points listing the key benefits or features of the product or service. For instance, the value proposition for the Thrifty White Pharmacy's Synchronized Medication Refill Program consists of:

1. *(A headline)* SIMPLIFY YOUR LIFE. SYNCHRONIZED MEDICATION REFILL PROGRAM

2. *(A short 2 to 3 sentence paragraph explaining what is offered, for whom and why is it useful)* THE PHARMACY WILL CONTACT YOU WHEN YOU NEED YOUR PRESCRIPTIONS FILLED. YOUR PHARMACIST WILL CHECK FOR CHANGES IN THERAPY AND POSSIBLE DRUG INTERACTIONS. BEST OF ALL, YOU WILL HAVE TIME TO TALK TO YOUR PHARMACIST AND ASK ANY QUESTIONS ABOUT YOUR MEDICATIONS.

3. *(Bullet points listing benefits and/or features)*
   - NO NEED TO CALL IN PRESCRIPTION REFILLS
   - FEWER TRIPS TO THE PHARMACY
   - NO WORRIES ABOUT RUNNING OUT OF YOUR MEDICINE

The basic points in Thrifty White's value proposition for its program are repeated in messaging for all promotional channels. This includes the company's website, Youtube videos, public relations efforts, store signage, and face-to-face conversations with patients.

Value propositions in community pharmacy settings can contain economic, functional, emotional, or symbolic appeals.[3] Most revolve around economic appeals like saving money and functional appeals like one-stop shopping, fast service, and easy in-and-out. This is reasonable because these are the value propositions expected by customers. However, pharmacists should experiment with emotional and symbolic propositions to tap into other patient values.[4]

Emotional value propositions center on feelings associated with the service experience or act of shopping (e.g., "You deserve some 'me time'. Stop by our cosmetics counter for a free makeover."). Emotional appeals can tap into connections between pharmacies and their customers because pharmacists are an important part of many patients' lives. They are friends, confidants, coaches, protectors, and more.

The success of emotional value propositions relies on their ability to make people feel something during their pharmacy experience.[4] For example, they might elicit the following responses, "When I visit Johnson's Apothecary, I feel - ___."

- protected from harm
- like part of the community
- like the pharmacist really cares about me as a person
- like I am revisiting my childhood

A visit to the pharmacist can have symbolic meaning too. The act of patronizing one pharmacy instead of another can be seen by people a way of expressing their values. For example, a customer who drives past a WalMart Megastore to visit a local independently owned pharmacy may do so to express support for local businesses. A person may visit a Pharmaca Integrative Pharmacy, which offer traditional pharmacy services alongside holistic remedies, to express feelings of being natural, in harmony with nature, stress-free, and other symbolic meanings.

Successful symbolic value propositions reinforce messages about what it says about a person who shops at a specific pharmacy. Statements of self-expression do not need to be around health either. They can be self-expressive benefits of being cool, cutting edge, technologically adept, or any other expression. For instance, they might elicit the following self-expressions, "When I visit my Pharmaca Pharmacy, I am____."

- o showing how smart I am about my health
- o demonstrating that I care about the environment
- o letting everyone know that I care about my family

SERVICE ADVERTISING STRATEGIES

Some marketers argue that different strategies should be used for advertising services than for promoting merchandise.[5] It is relatively simple to advertise tangible objects like automobiles, food, and other consumer products because can be easily represented in pictures or verbal descriptions. Services are less easy to promote because they are intangible performances that are difficult to visualize and understand. For instance, how does one characterize MTM services in an image or words that are meaningful and easy to understand?

Television news broadcasts often attempt to illustrate pharmacist services by linking pharmacists to something tangible. News stories about pharmacy typically show pharmacists counting tablets on a tray. The tablets are a convenient prop for letting viewers know that this is a pharmacist and not someone else. Without seeing the tablets, viewers might not recognize the person as a pharmacist. The problem is that counting tablets is not really an accurate depiction of what pharmacists do.

The unique characteristics of services, such as intangibility and inconsistency, make it difficult to convey meaningful messages about services in advertising. Marketers have suggested various strategies to overcome the limitations of services to make them more visually meaningful (Table 15-1).[5-7]

One strategy is to make services more tangible in ads. This might be achieved through images of physical facilities or use of concrete symbols or language. Seeing the counseling or drive-through area of a pharmacy gives consumers context for thinking about the service experience. Such images attempt to relate an abstract concept (i.e., a service) to a tangible one (i.e., an object). Tangible objects associated with pharmacy services include computers, telephones, prescription bottles, and company logos. Even a picture of a smiling pharmacist can be used. The mortar and pestle, a symbol of pharmacy's past, is still seen.

Table 15-1 Strategies to Overcome Problems with Advertising Pharmacy Services

Problem	Strategies
Services are intangible. Accordingly, services are more difficult to grasp conceptually.	-Make pharmaceutical services more tangible in the advertisement. -Incorporate physical elements of the service into the advertisement. -Show a picture of the counseling area or the drive-through pharmacy. -Associate the service with a concrete symbol.
Services are inseparable from their production and consumption. Services often require the presence and participation of the customer.	-Demonstrate the patient's participation. -Show the pharmacist and patient together in the advertisement. -Show the patient accessing pharmacist services by telephone or Internet.
Services are heterogeneous; no two service experiences are alike. Excellent service one day may be replaced by a horrible experience the next day.	-Use documentation of the consistent high quality of pharmacist services. -Include results of satisfaction surveys or Gallup Polls in the ad. -Display achievements such as certification as a diabetes educator or as a Verified Internet Pharmacy Practice Site. -Simulate word-of-mouth recommendations with a testimonial from a customer about excellent service.
The service experience is difficult for consumers to visualize.	-Show the service experience as a series of events. -Illustrate superior pharmacy service in a television advertisement (e.g., when a pharmacist prevented a serious drug reaction). -Include text that shows the simple steps involved in completing a telephone refill.

Sources: [5-7]

☐

Another strategy is to make the relationship between the consumer and the provider explicit in the advertisement. Many pharmacy ads show a patient and a pharmacist consulting about medications. This gives consumers a clearer image of the service. Other ads show consumers speaking on the telephone (presumably to the pharmacy) or contacting pharmacies by Internet.

Documentation can be used in advertisements to underscore the quality and value of services. Using documented measures of quality helps differentiate one service provider from the next. Advertisements can highlight customer satisfaction scores or special awards for exemplary services. The Verified Internet Pharmacy Practice Site seal is awarded by the National Association of Boards of Pharmacy to Internet pharmacy sites that meet certain requirements. Consumers can use this symbol to identify quality Internet pharmacies.

Another way of emphasizing the quality and value of services in ads is to simulate word-of-mouth recommendations by showing people discussing the services. This can be accomplished by having customers, real or simulated, talk about previous service experiences. Sometimes celebrity spokespersons are used. It is important that the celebrity in advertisements be seen as credible, likable, and representative of the image promoted by the marketer.

Finally, the steps involved in the service experience itself can be illustrated in advertising text or images. A visit to a pharmacy might be illustrated with a series of images showing a pharmacist receiving a prescription, checking the patient profile, calling the physician to verify information, and then giving the patient the medication, along with counseling.

3. SELECT AN INTEGRATED COMMUNICATION MIX

Rarely do pharmacists use just one promotional channel to get their message to customers and stakeholders. Instead they may post signs, put flyers in customers' bags, use social media, hold public relations events, or just talk to customers. It is important that communications be integrated in a consistent and reinforcing way. The effectiveness of a communication mix is defined by the following equation:

$$\text{Message Effectiveness} = \text{Reach} \times \text{Frequency} \times \text{Relevance}$$

A marketing communication's effectiveness is determined by the messages *reach* (total number of different individuals exposed to a message), *frequency* (number to times that each individual is exposed to the message), and *relevancy* (importance of the communication to each individual at the time and context of exposure). The use of multiple methods increases the message's reach by giving individuals multiple opportunities to be exposed to it. Not all people read the newspaper, listen to the radio, are connected to the Internet, and watch television, but most people take part in at least one of these activities.

Multiple methods also increase the opportunities to be exposed to messages more times, in more ways, and in different times and contexts. Repeated exposures to messages using diverse forms of media can increase the opportunity for them to be noticed and remembered. The variety of ways in which individuals are exposed also allows the message to reach individuals at various stages of the pharmacy experience. A television advertisement can increase awareness of pharmacy services, a coupon can get a consumer to visit a pharmacy, and a pharmacist can personally sell the value of a needed professional service. When these messages work together in a consistent, integrated manner, they can more effectively achieve desired communication objectives.

The selection of media depends on the budget for promotional communications and which promotional media will be most efficient and effective in influencing target customers. A rule of thumb is that the cost increases as more people are reached with the marketing message and as the message is more personalized.

However, promotions on the Internet seem to break this rule, since it is possible to send a message on the Web to millions of people for very little money. A promotional message in a blog, video clip, or e-mail can spread like a virus through professional and social Web networks; this is an inexpensive means of making an exponential impact on thoughts and behaviors. The right message at the right time in the right way can spread rapidly across the world.

> A brand is no longer what we tell the consumer it is. It is what consumers tell each other it is.
>
> — Scott Cook, Founder of Intuit

Promoting Buzz

Buzz or word-of-mouth marketing is a set of strategies to get others to spread a marketer's message. Pharmacists can best promote buzz about their products and services as part of an integrated communication strategy, incorporating advertising and other techniques that reinforce and support each other. There are seven steps associated with a buzz marketing strategy:[8]

1. **Choose a buzzworthy idea.** A buzz-worthy idea must be innovative, personally relevant, and clearly superior to what is currently available. Visible and tangible objects are more likely to generate conversation. An interesting story will make the idea more likely to be recalled and shared with others. A life-saving drug discovered in an Amazon rain forest or at the bottom of an ocean will generate buzz better than a new drug insurance plan.

2. **Identify opinion leaders among the group you wish to influence**. Opinion leaders have greater influence on the spread of ideas because they are "connected"; they readily interact with others by nature or through their work. They are up-to-date with new trends and freely express their views. They may feel and act differently from others and be more likely to rebel against the status quo.

3. **Approach opinion leaders in a way that gets them talking**. People talk about the extraordinary, not the commonplace. Thus, buzz is driven by the marketer's imagination; a quirky advertisement or outrageous promotional stunt can help spread buzz about a product. Controversy can generate buzz, and so can extremes (e.g., top 10 or worst 5 lists). Some marketers generate buzz by promoting the existence of a "secret" and making people guess what it is. Sometimes an object or idea itself is sufficient to get people talking, particularly if the marketer provides samples or a demonstration.

4. **Identify and overcome obstacles and bottlenecks to adoption**. Buzz can be stopped at any time in its early development. Negative word-of-mouth caused by an unmet expectation or bad experience can halt buzz in its tracks. Marketers must continually assess peoples' experience with innovations to determine the degree to which they meet expectations and needs. Problems with the product itself should be resolved immediately. Any systemic barriers that could hamper adoption should be identified and addressed.

5. **Use different channels of communication**. Buzz marketing is typically integrated with other promotional communications. Combining buzz with other methods can broaden the reach and effectiveness of promotional messages.

6. **Encourage adaptation**. If an innovation is not used exactly as it was originally designed, that is OK. Adaptation of innovations to new situations is common; it should be encouraged because it helps facilitate adoption. Adaptation works best when individuals use innovations to resolve their own needs, and not necessarily the needs intended by marketers.

7. **Ask for an endorsement**. Once opinion leaders have adopted an innovation, get their endorsement. Have them comment on the innovation, and get permission to quote them in promotional fliers and advertisements. Encourage them to tell others about the benefits of the innovation. If they willingly champion the innovation, get permission to refer others to them to hear about their experience.

Like all third party marketing methods, buzz marketing has downsides. Buzz can be negative as well as positive. It turns negative if it stimulates demand that outstrips supply and customers become frustrated. Furthermore, buzz marketing can backfire if it leads consumers to feel deceived or manipulated by marketers. Some buzz marketing firms have misrepresented paid marketing as spontaneous word-of-mouth; they have paid "shoppers" to visit Web sites or trendy locations and rave about products. Buzz marketers have also paid for ghost-written promotional pieces and represented them as unbiased work.

Deceptive buzz tactics can destroy the credibility of marketing messages and make consumers even more cynical and suspicious toward marketers. Pharmacists should use buzz sparingly and cautiously. A poorly planned and initiated campaign can damage consumers' confidence in pharmacists and the perception of pharmacists as credible advocates for patients.

INTEGRATED MESSAGING THROUGHOUT THE CUSTOMER JOURNEY

Chapter 11 on consumer behavior describes how marketers view the consumer decision process as a journey. Throughout the journey, customers interact with the provider at numerous touchpoints - each an opportunity to communicate an integrated message. Therefore, mapping the various touchpoints in the journey will help identify where communications can occur and what they should say.

For example, Figure 15-2 shows the customer journey with an appointment based medication synchronization program (ABMS). This customer journey map breaks the experience into before, during, and after stages of the journey. Within each stage, distinct experiences occur with the service provider. These are labeled experiences because they describe what the customer sees and experiences, not what the pharmacist communicates. In the end, it does not matter what the pharmacist says or does - only what the customer perceives.

To illustrate, the customer journey map shows that face-to-face discussions between with pharmacy personnel and patients is key to most stages of the customer ABMS journey. They are important in helping patients learn details about the ABMS Program, the signing of the contract, the effectiveness of the monthly, the appointment itself, and whether the patient continues with the program or not. Knowing this and consciously planning communication messaging from employees can help integrate communications about the program.

Several suggestions can help pharmacists use the customer journey to select an integrated communication mix. One is to map out and study the whole customer journey to identify the contexts in which customers interact with the pharmacy, products, or services. These contexts include face-to-face, web, phone call, social media, and even the pharmacy's parking lot experiences. Then pharmacists should choose only a limited number (two or three) experiences to focus on. With each experience, one should define what would be a successful outcome. For instance, a successful phone call might be one in which the caller feels like they been treated in a respectful, friendly manner. An experience with a pharmacy parking lot is one where the customer feels welcomed to enter. After that, look at the current customer experience from the patient's viewpoint. Call the pharmacy or have someone else call and assess the experience. Drive into the parking lot like you have never been there and note what you see or how you feel. Based upon your experiences, make a change.

Figure 15-2 Customer Journey with an Appointment-Based Medication Synchronization Program (ABMS)

	Before		During					After	
	Patient (pt) goes to the pharmacy	Pt learns details of ABMS Program	Pt signs ABMS contract	Pt brings Rxs to pharmacy to choose synch date	Monthly call prior to picking up the meds	Pt appt. to pick up meds	RPh speaks with pt about issues	Pt persists with ABMS or not	Pt talks of ABMS to others
Experience with upfront pharmacy experience	X								
Website Experience	X								
Experience with POS signage and other messaging		X							
Experience with basic dispensing experience								X	
Word-of-mouth experiences from other customers	X	X							
Word-of-mouth recommendations from health care professionals			X					X	
Face-to-face discussions with pharmacy personnel		X	X	X		X	X	X	X
Experience with Phone calls		X			X			X	
Experience with Social media									

4. ASSESS THE EFFECTIVENESS OF THE COMMUNICATIONS

In designing promotional plans, it is important to define success by some objective measure. There is no way to know if promotional communications are successful until their results are measured. There are many ways to measure the success of marketing communications including the following:

- Examining changes in sales after promotional events,

- Asking new customers how they heard about your business,

- Asking patients if they remember seeing your mailed brochure and if they can describe what it said, and

- Observing whether consumer behavior changes; for example, did a patient who was enrolled in a smoking cessation program stop smoking?

Measures of promotional effectiveness should be chosen before any strategies are implemented. They should not be completed as an afterthought. In fact, knowing what you want your communications are expected to achieve beforehand can help when crafting the messaging. This sounds like common sense, but many communication plans do not always have a clear outcome in mind.

5. CONDUCT A PROMOTIONAL COMMUNICATIONS AUDIT

Pharmacies communicate through a variety of channels -- conversations with patients, newspaper circulars, shelf stickers, signage, mailing, radio advertising, coupons, and more. Communications audits can assess whether messaging is unified across all channels -- providing a consistent and reinforced message centered on the strategic plan.

A communications audit is a systematic assessment of a business's promotional practices with the purpose of gaining a clear depiction of current strategy and actions. The goal is to identify what works well, what needs to be improved, and what adjustments might occur. For example, a communications audit of a medication therapy management program in a single Walgreens or CVS store needs to evaluate both the store's communications strategy and the chain's strategy for consistency and coherence. If the store's communications conflict with the chain's, dissonance may occur in the mind of the patient about the chain's brand.

An audit consists of a list of all of the communications produced by the pharmacy. This list can be developed in conjunction with a customer journey map.

After compiling the list, details can be added like the specific audiences targeted with the communications, the primary message to be conveyed or experienced, and the desired outcome. This information can be organized into a table like the one illustrated in Table 15-3 to allow comparisons of channel messaging and outcomes.

Table 15-3 Example of a communications audit

Communication channel	Target audience(s) (can be > 1)	How does exposure occur?	Primary message	Desired outcome
Coupon	Price conscious patients, senior citizens	Newspaper circular, pharmacy website, direct mail, Facebook, Twitter	Buy this now or soon	Purchase Phazyme (relieve your gas)
TV ad	Busy patients, patients over 45 years of age	Television, possibly Youtube	You are busy & we can help	Consider using us to help you manage your busy life
Public sign	One-stop shoppers, commuters	Local Billboard	We are convenient	A visit to the pharmacy to shop

The audit can help the overall messaging strategy by answering the following questions:

1. What is the message being sent by the channels? Is that the message which was desired?
2. How coherent and consistent is that message?
3. Which of the communications channels is most (and least) effective? Why?
4. Which of the communications messages is most (and least) effective? Why?
5. Which communications are inconsistent with the overall message sent by the channels?
6. What communication channel is underutilized or not used?
7. What communication channel is not providing enough value for its cost?

MARKETING IN ACTION

Assessing the Impact of a Promotional Effort

Familiprix, a mid-size regional drugstore chain in Quebec, Canada implemented a promotional campaign in 2002 to respond to pressures from its primary competitors: Jean Coutu and Pharmaprix (the Shoppers Drug Mart in Quebec). Familiprix found that top-of-mind awareness (i.e., % of respondents who mentioned Familiprix when asked to list local pharmacies) for the Familiprix brand was only 19%, compared to 90+% for Jean Coutu and 60+% for Pharmaprix. In addition, the Familiprix name was regularly confused with Pharmaprix and Uniprix (other mid-sized chains).

Familiprix set an objective to keep health-related sales growing by 15% over the next 6-month period and increase top-of-mind awareness by 10%. They planned on achieving the objective by increasing their focus on health-related products/nonprescription drugs and targeting promotional efforts on young families with kids. In addition, they broadcasted a humorous television advertising campaign.

Only three weeks after launch of the promotional campaign, Familiprix's top-of-mind awareness jumped from 19% to 37%. By the end of the year, it was an amazing 52%; an increase of 33 points (remember that their goal was only 10%). Sales of health-related products also grew 33% versus an objective of +15%.

The success of the marketing campaign was attributed primarily to the humorous TV commercials where the Canadian actor Sylvain Marcel played a pharmacist in a white lab coat. Blending into everyday situations, he would appear and suddenly yell "Ah-ha! Familiprix!" when it was obvious that the help of a pharmacist was needed. Situations included a shopper who bangs herself against a window, an ex-smoker bumming a cigarette, and a young couple, home alone for the week-end. Like 'Where's the Beef ' and 'Whasuuuuuuup,' the 'Ah Ha Familiprix' line became a popular culture phenomenon.

Source: Reference[9]

SUMMARY

All pharmacists engage in marketing communication. Some do so better than others. The key is to thoughtfully develop and implement a communications plan that follows the steps and strategies described in this chapter. These can help pharmacists be more effective in achieving their goals and avoiding common blunders.

Reference List

(1) Berkowitz J. A hosptial rebrands chemotherapy with the help of superheros. Fast Company [June]. 2013. 6-3-2013.

(2) Laja P. Useful value propositions examples (and how to create one). 2-16-2012. 2-6-2015.

(3) Sorescu A, Frambach RT, Singh J, Rangaswamy A, Bridges C. Innovations in Retail Business Models. Journal of Retailing 2011;87, Supplement 1(0):S3-S16.

(4) Aaker D. Beyond functional benefits. Marketing news 2009;43:23.

(5) Zeithaml VA, Parasuraman A, Berry LL. Problems and Strategies in Services Marketing. Journal of Marketing 1985;49(Spring):33-46.

(6) Zeithaml VA, MJ. B. Services Marketing. 1st ed. New York: McGraw-Hill Companies Inc.; 1996.

(7) Holdford D, Yom SH. Content analysis of newspaper advertising of pharmacy services. Journal of Pharmaceutical Marketing & Management 2003;15(2):81-96.

(8) Holdford DA. Using buzz marketing to promote ideas, services, and products. Journal of the American Pharmacists Association: JAPhA 2003;44(3):387-395.

(9) Rhéaume A., Bernier J., Fabien M, Courtois M., Moreau J. Familiprix: Case Study. Warc com 2005; Available at: URL: http://www.warc.com/Search/ Familiprix/Familiprix.warc?q= Familiprix &Area=CaseStudies&Tab=.

Chapter Questions

1. Visit a local pharmacy. Walk though the store and talk to employees. Visit the pharmacy's website too. Based upon your experience, develop a positioning strategy statement for the pharmacy based upon your experience and the messaging of the store.

2. Look at a service being promoted at a pharmacy website. Identify the value proposition being communicated for that service. Who is the primary audience for this value proposition? What is the problem (or problems) faced by customers for which the service offers a solution? What are the main features of the product or service to be provided? How does it compare with what is currently in the marketplace? What evidence or proof points are offered to support the value proposition?

3. View a TV, newspaper, Internet, or other advertisement promoting a pharmacist delivered service. Identify what strategies from Table 15-2 are used to advertise these services.

4. Discuss if MTM services are buzzworthy? How might buzz about MTM services be promoted in a manner that is ethical and professional?

5. Choose a major pharmacy chain. Identify all of the ways the chain uses social media marketing. Discuss the relative effectiveness of each.

INDEX

Note: Capitalized Words are Headings of Sections

Made in the USA
Middletown, DE
23 August 2016